Understanding Arthritis—The Clinical Way Forward

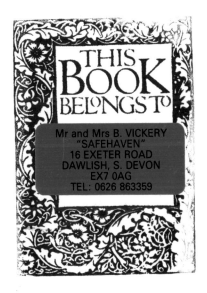

Understanding Arthritis

The Clinical Way Forward

William W. Fox, MB, MRCS

and

David L. J. Freed, MD

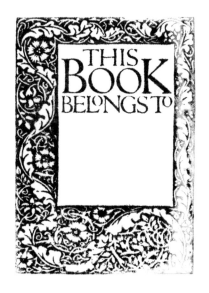

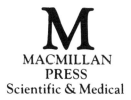

MACMILLAN
PRESS
Scientific & Medical

First published 1990

Published by
THE MACMILLAN PRESS LTD
Houndmills, Basingstoke, Hampshire RG21 2XS
and London
Companies and representatives
throughout the world

Filmset by Wearside Tradespools
Fulwell, Sunderland

Printed in Hong Kong

British Library Cataloguing in Publication Data
Fox, William W. (William Woolfe), 1905–
Understanding arthritis.
1. Man. Rheumatic diseases. Joints. Arthritis. Arthritis &
rheumatic diseases
I. Title.   II. Freed, David L. J.
616.7'2
ISBN 0–333–44440–X
      0–333–53413–1 (pb)

Contents

Preface

Not so long ago, in the medical world, the word 'flux' (diarrhoea) was considered to be a diagnosis. The patient had a flux, the remedy was so-and-so. Nowadays, of course, doctors recognise many different causes of diarrhoea, and cannot be satisfied with that simple descriptive label because the different varieties of diarrhoea demand quite different treatments. Diarrhoea caused by ulcerative colitis might very well be treated with steroid enemas, whereas the same treatment for an infection of the bowel would be catastrophic. The science of microbiology — the outstanding example of how examination of the environment can revolutionise the management of real-life illness in humans — has taught us to distinguish carefully between the different causes of a symptom and to make what is called an **aetiological diagnosis**, that is, a diagnosis that includes an identification of the cause.

Once upon a time physicians recognised an entity called consumption, or phthisis. It was a recognisable group of symptoms and signs that occurred again and again in different patients, that is, a **syndrome**. It was an entity, a disease, an attacker on the body. Along came Robert Koch, a brilliant nineteenth-century scientist, and in an epic adventure of science taking up many years he tracked down 'the cause' — a germ called *Mycobacterium tuberculosis*. Koch discovered a simple method for finding the germ in patients' sputum, or in the tissues, and virtually overnight physicians stopped talking about consumption and phthisis. Today's medical students have never heard the words. Instead, medicine had a brand-new disease called tuberculosis, which eventually led to new methods of treatment which have virtually eradicated the disease from the Western world.

However, today's doctors still fail, very often, to learn the lesson of nineteenth-century microbiology. We still too often talk about 'asthma', 'migraine' and 'arthritis' as if these words were diagnoses. They are not. They are descriptive labels, just like flux and phthisis. They are the first stage towards making a diagnosis, the identification of a syndrome. The words do not tell us the causes. The body has only a limited repertoire of symptoms and signs. The skin can produce a rash called eczema, for example, which can be caused by dozens of different things. The same is true of asthma, migraine and arthritis. The word 'arthritis' means no more than 'inflammation of the joint(s)', and even that is often a misnomer, as we shall see below.

I have known Dr. Bill Fox since 1979, and respect him as a fellow scientist. Many others fail to realise how much a scientist he is because he is unfamiliar with modern conventional scientists' rhetoric. He was trained as a doctor nearly 60 years ago, and his style of expression and writing is that of the doctors of those days. Many professional scientists of today will read his portion of this book with disdain because of the style in which it is couched, but scientist he is. He looks at patients and listens carefully to what they say. He finds much of what they say inexplicable, and sets out to search for more satisfying explanations of what he sees. He erects hypotheses, and then tests them against the realities of clinical life. His experiments have led him to a conclusion — although he recognises, as all good scientists do, that there is no such thing as the ultimate 'truth' in science, that there is always much more to be understood — that much of the chronic ill health seen in general practice, adorned with a multitude of symptoms and descriptive medical epithets, is caused by the slow, chronic, rheumatic process that he describes. His view may or may not be correct, or it may turn out to be partially correct. Like all good medical hypotheses, it is testable and it leads on to predictions as to the types of treatment that might be most (and least) appropriate. Bill Fox is now nearing the end of his active life; it is up to other scientists and doctors to take up the baton that he is holding out.

It should be understood that the claims he makes about the treatment, based on this hypothesis, are in no way exaggerated. I personally have seen about 50 of his patients over the last nine years. Because of the accumulated evidence of his excellent success rate, I have recently started to use his methods in my own practice, with equally satisfactory results.

No medical innovator is thanked by his peers — totally new insights in medicine are uncomfortable to doctors as they carry the implication that up until this point we were all doing things wrong. Medical innovators are always greeted with hostility by their fellow medics. This has been Bill Fox's experience also, but he may take comfort from two reflections:

1. Although unpopular, his work has always followed the principles of the greatest teachers of mainstream orthodox medicine.
2. He is neither the first nor the last medical innovator to be scorned by his peers during his lifetime.

However, if there is any truth at all in his beliefs, if he has come even a little closer to the ultimate truth than others have done, he will receive his recognition one day, and will have brought untold and untellable benefit to suffering human beings.

This book is Bill Fox's account of the rheumatic patch, which is an important contributory factor in the chronic rheumatic diseases but which is ignored by most medical textbooks. He reports how he discovered rheumatic patches, and learned their importance and how to treat them effectively, with results so good and so fast that most doctors who witness the treatment have difficulty in believing their eyes. He also tells of his parallel discoveries: the importance of commensal diphtheroids in the throat, and the usefulness of antihistamines. My part, as an academic immunologist and also Bill Fox's pupil in clinical rheumatology, is to provide (as far as possible) a scientific interpretation of his clinical findings.

Rheumatic disease causes an enormous load of human misery, as well as a quite shocking death rate [1], both from the disease itself and from the drugs used to alleviate its effects [2]. History will not readily forgive the medical profession, if in our caution or our conservatism we fail to examine carefully every possibility of effective drugless treatments, even though the ideas might be novel.

University of Salford, 1989   D.L.J.F.

Prologue

I qualified as a doctor in 1929. After two years in hospital and locum work I entered general practice. Within a further two years it became abundantly clear that my ability to diagnose, treat or refer patients (excluding the infectious diseases) was restricted to about 20 cases per annum. These represented the major diseases which filled the textbooks and the patients who occupied the beds in the teaching hospitals.

The vast majority of the patients in general practice complained of vague aches and pains or discomfort designated according to their location, such as headaches, migraine, stiff necks, brachial neuralgia, pleurodynia, lumbago, sciatica coxalgia, slipped disc, cramp in the hands or feet, undiagnosable pains or discomfort in the chest or abdomen. Sore throats and 'colds', loss of energy and depression frequently accompanied many of these symptoms. Finally there were the cases of proven (by X-ray) osteo- and rheumatoid arthritis.

The great value of our hospital training was not so much the diagnosis of the major diseases, but the insistence on a meticulous attention to every detail of the patient's history and symptoms and the absolute requirement of a thorough physical examination of the patient. It was in this way that our great clinical masters of the past were able to present to us complete detailed analyses of diseases which provided the sure foundations of understanding and diagnosis on which modern scientific medicine could be applied to find a cure for so many complaints. This was the dilemma which confronted me in the 1930s.

A diagnosis could be achieved in only a limited number of cases. The remainder were conglomerations of symptoms which had no meaning, no understanding and could therefore be treated symptomatically only, which is about as unscientific as one can get. I therefore resolved to pay meticulous attention to all of these cases. Slowly and arduously I began to perceive a hazy relationship between all those symptoms listed earlier—they seemed to be interwoven into a rheumatic pattern. So I decided that I must study the chronic rheumatic diseases.

To this end I moved to London, took on a small general practice and became a clinical assistant at the Charterhouse Rheumatism Clinic and also, because I had studied some osteopathy, clinical assistant to Mr. W. E. Tucker in the Orthopaedic Department of the Royal London Homeopathic Hospital.

Treatment at the Charterhouse consisted of a vaccine made from a number of organisms isolated from the throats of rheumatic patients by its founder, Dr. Warren-Crowe. Physical medicine and later gold were introduced. Within a year or so, I formed the opinion that the value of the treatment was questionable. I began to wonder what I was doing there and thought of resigning. In a moment of blinding lucidity I realised that this was the heaven-sent opportunity I wanted — to study the natural history of the chronic rheumatic diseases.

During the war the Honorary President of the Charterhouse Clinic, the Duchess of Kent, opened the new clinic in Weymouth Street and just prior to that I became a Consultant.

What I chronicled during the next 12 years was published in 1950 [3] and formed the basis of all my researches since then. Re-reading what was written there, I see its deficiencies in the light of modern attitudes, but its essential clinical truth survives and holds its place in the basic diagnostic criteria required in the understanding of the chronic rheumatic diseases. Four years after publication of this paper there was no point in remaining at the Charterhouse.

I later made contact with Mr. Tucker who had spent many years in the army. He suffered from osteoarthritis of both hips and I suggested he might like to try the effects of injecting some rheumatic patches. He readily agreed and was so impressed with the result that he asked me to return as Clinical Collaborator in the Orthopaedic Department at the Royal London Homeopathic Hospital. Following this my study of osteoarthritis of the hip was published.

Unfortunately Bill Tucker retired and so my association with the hospital was terminated. He suggested I went to America with him to open a clinic, but I declined because I did not feel that the problems were properly solved, and there was more research needed. However, in 1983, a doctor whom I trained became a visiting consultant at the hospital in Bermuda, which was part of the Tucker territory.

My studies at the Charterhouse Clinic showed quite clearly that patients slowly but surely deteriorated, with occasional remission of their symptoms which could last from a few weeks to up to two years. Relapses were sudden with an acute exacerbation of one area, or an entirely new part of the body, and they were frequently heralded by a feeling of malaise and a mild sore throat.

In a clinic of 50 patients, if one presented with this story you could be quite sure there would be at least five others by the end of the session. This was a clinical reinforcement of the possibility of a viral infection.

Furthermore, it was obvious that patients got used to a lower standard of health and function and a greater tolerance of pain, so that any judgement of minor improvement in the reduction of swelling or pain, or slight increase of function attributed to drugs or physical medicine, must remain suspect. The only drug that would produce a clear impression of improvement is a steroid but this is a drug which flatters to deceive, and one which I would never use.

The essential basis of the treatment is to inject the appropriate rheumatic patches with 0.5% solution of sodium salicylate. This will produce an almost immediate response in diminution of pain and increased movement. For example, in osteoarthritis of the hip the patient will be able to raise himself from a chair more easily, followed by increased ability in walking and weight bearing, especially to be noted in dealing with staircases. In the same way, loss of movement and power in rheumatoid arthritis can be improved with a resultant stronger and less painful grip.

For all these reasons, I insist that my treatment must produce an unequivocal improvement within two or three minutes, that it is repeatable and does not require any anti-rheumatic drugs or pain killers except a limited use of aspirin. That is why I claim immediate improvement in at least 80% of all cases treated—a figure which is corroborated by a rheumatologist in Bulgaria where similar treatment is available in every district hospital for osteoarthrosis [4].

Some five years ago I conducted a private seminar at the house of Professor Eli Davis in Jerusalem. In his concluding remarks he said how very impressed he was with my presentation, but found great difficulty in believing me because my claim for improvements was so high—if it had been around 50% he would have accepted it!

My reply was rhetorical: 'Do you want me to tell lies so that you should believe me?' Read this book and decide for yourself.

London, September 1989   W.W.F.

CHAPTER 1

Introduction

It was in 1926 that all of us who had survived the *pons asinorum* of anatomy and physiology attended our first lecture in medicine.

The professor told us how privileged we were to become members of the most noble profession in the world because, in conquering disease, we were destined to cause our own destruction! As he said this, I vividly remember thinking 'My goodness, I hope this doesn't happen before we're qualified!' Ignorance, naiveté and a lurking sense of humour were all inextricably mingled in that thought. With experience of life as it really is, and the widespread problems of sickness which were encountered in general practice, I began to understand the euphoria of our professor. His world was bounded by the hospital and consulting room, where only major diseases were admitted. At that time, insulin had just been discovered. Anaesthetics (ether and chloroform) were making more operations possible and the surgical attack on cancer was going to eradicate that killer! So here were two major diseases ready for elimination. The remainder would surely follow.

Well, it has not turned out quite like that. Diabetic treatment has improved but there is no cure. Surgical treatment of cancer has been improved by restricting the surgical excesses of yesteryear and the addition of X-ray treatment, laser techniques and chemotherapy.

So the euphoria of pie in the sky continued. This was significantly bolstered—not without good reason—when antibiotics were discovered. As we all know, their undoubted benefits (I would not be alive today without them) have been followed by the emergence of resistant strains, and serious new diseases such as legionnaires' disease and AIDS.

Also, surgical techniques have made immense strides in the treatment of serious injuries, transplants, and replacement techniques, including test-tube babies. Once again, the euphoria is stimulated. All these remarkable achievements hold the promise that the scientific pursuit of all the medical problems will be solved in due time.

From the viewpoint of the consultants in their hospitals, this seems reasonable. However, from the viewpoint of a general practitioner, as I used to be, no progress whatsoever is seen in the treatment of that persistent mass of ill health which crowds the doctors' waiting rooms and hospitals, precisely because clinical medicine has made no progress in recognising or understanding what they are. There are no diagnoses, only names, such as headaches, migraine, torticollis, a whole variety of neuralgias and backaches, tennis elbow, strained ligaments and muscles—the list is endless. There are also those indeterminate pains in the chest and abdomen for which they cannot even think of a name, much less a diagnosis. Some of these become categorised as the tensions, the neurotics and the malingerers. Because I have never believed that people want to be ill, I have tried to understand their complaints by listening, questioning and examining. That is how I came to learn so much of the early and natural history of the chronic rheumatic diseases and somehow perceived a vague relationship between them and that endless list of complaints.

Let us spend a moment in analysing this problem.

In the case of pneumonia cured by an antibiotic, we know everything about the diagnosis, the pathology and the cause of the disease—a pneumococcus. Science produced a specific cure—an antibiotic which would destroy the germ. Now consider a stone impacted in the ureter. We are not certain of the cause, but we do know every clinical detail which will enable us to make a precise diagnosis. Science is then enlisted to confirm the diagnosis with X-rays, and to provide instruments and laser beams to break up the stone into dust without damaging the ureter, and so the stone is passed painlessly out of the bladder in the urine.

Now consider rheumatoid arthritis. The cause remains unknown, the onset of the disease is not recognised and an arbitrary line is drawn when the disease is accepted as a diagnosis—there must be X-ray evidence of joint damage and a positive rheumatoid factor. All this is contrary to the basic science of clinical examination and diagnosis.

A study of the well-established clinical disease of measles is a model of how the diagnosis is established from the incubation period followed by chronological details of all the symptoms: temperature; running eyes and nose; photophobia; Koplik's spots; the rash starting on the face and spreading down the body; the details of the rash itself and finally the resolution of the disease. This is a comprehensive intelligible picture which enables you to suspect its onset in the very early stages.

In contrast with the 3–4 weeks of this disease, let us look at syphilis. In syphilis, a chancre develops within a week of infection. This is followed by enlarged inguinal glands. Six weeks later a rash develops over the body and gradually gets better. Ten or twenty years later gummas may develop in various viscera, and much later than that tabes dorsalis or GPI make their appearance. In addition, an infected female will have several stillbirths.

Is it not remarkable that without any scientific help whatsoever clinicians were able to construct a clinical picture spread over almost a lifetime?

What we should learn from these examples is that the science of clinicial diagnosis, which means clinical understanding of the disease, is a basic priority to the use of any other science.

May I put it quite simply: when science is the handmaiden to the clinical masters, their services are assessable and justly rewarded, but when the handmaid becomes the mistress of the 'clinical masters' then the services become outrageously expensive and inevitably much less rewarding. Sadly, this is the present situation with chronic rheumatic disease and that vast mass of ill health referred to earlier.

Here is a recent example, related to my paper presented on 'the rheumatic patch' at an international seminar on rheumatic diseases in 1987 [12]. It appeared to be very well received and the next speaker, Dr. Bitnum, prefaced his paper by saying that my presentation was so good that it made me a very difficult man to follow and that at future meetings he would try to speak before me! He then read his paper on hip pain in children [5].

There were 21 cases, aged from 2 to 12. After listing all the possible causes, his analysis of examination was as follows:

In 86% one hip was affected, in 14% both.
In 20% there was definite reduction in the range of movement.
In 30% no objective signs were present.
In 60% the diagnosis was transient synovitis.
In 25% the diagnosis was arthralgia, cause unknown.
The average duration of pain was 18 days.
90% were managed at home.
Over 50% had various blood tests done.
33% had X-rays.
There were follow-ups at 3 and 6 months.

His summary stated that almost all children with hip pain had an excellent prognosis and previous anxiety about further disease was no longer appropriate.

This is an example of modern scientific investigation. Compare this with a purely clinical examination carried out by me in scores of children during 40 years in general practice. A small number were very acute and raised the question of acute osteomyelitis, requiring bed rest and observation. The majority were not acute but presented with some limping and pain of which the child complained. There was no case which could not be related to a recent infectious disease or a sore throat.

Examination, which included palpation, revealed the presence of one or two superficial areas of pain, which some years later were identified as rheumatic patches.

In the early years, I was not able to correlate the pain and loss of movement with the painful areas. To use words such as transient synovitis or arthralgia of unknown cause as a diagnosis is to me a travesty of clinical medicine.

One of the greatest teachers of clinical medicine I had the good fortune to have received some training from was Mr. A. M. Burgess, Professor of Surgery at the Manchester Royal Infirmary. His dictum was that you must make a diagnosis on all the relevant data obtained from a medical history and a full clinical examination. Woe betide you if you hazarded a diagnosis without clinical evidence. Only at this stage could you justify a request for laboratory and X-ray investigations which would either support or disprove the diagnosis.

Transient synovitis, excepting where X-ray evidence has suggested it, or arthralgia of unknown origin are not diagnoses; they are words like 'lumbago' or 'trapped nerves' which cannot be substantiated by any clinical findings. Subcutaneous areas of pain—rheumatic patches—can easily be determined on examination. Explaining and relating them to hip pain constitutes a logical orthodox progression in clinical studies.

This is the basis of my work. I was then able to point out to Dr. Bitnum that—had he known about the rheumatic patch—all his investigations would have been unnecessary, as would those of many other researchers in their field all over the world.

What is even more important is the fact that this hip or leg pain in children can be recognised as a clinically identifiable rheumatic condition, just as Koplik's spots are an early feature of measles. When a detailed clinical history of a rheumatoid arthritis is taken, it will almost always reveal a history of 'growing pains' in childhood.

In this way, we really are making progress in the clinical history and understanding of the chronic rheumatic diseases, thus following the pattern of the old clinical masters without whose diligence all the well-understood diseases of today would not have been illumined.

CHAPTER 2

A New Approach to Arthritis

INTRODUCTION (W.W.F.)

This treatise on the chronic rheumatic diseases summarises the results of over 40 years of clinical observation and examination which started in general practice and gradually became specialised.

My objectives in writing this book are as follows:

1. To give a panoramic view of the chronic rheumatic diseases as they begin in childhood (frequently) and progress to old age.
2. To demonstrate that in comprehending the progression of the disease it is possible to retard its development, and to diminish its ravages on the joints in over 80% of cases.
3. To dispense with many of the drugs and physiotherapeutic treatments in wide and common use today.
4. To indicate a new line of approach in the scientific investigation of these diseases.
5. To demonstrate that the superficial fascia has a much greater role in the control of the locomotor system than is generally supposed by the anatomy, orthopaedic, neurological and arthritis disciplines.

Two papers and an earlier book [3, 6, 7] together with subsequent findings over the last 10 years constitute the basis of this book.

In 1950 it seemed that the paradox confronting the study of the chronic rheumatic diseases was that, while their classification offered a wide variety of apparently unrelated, or distantly related, diseases, treatment was identical. It consisted of physiotherapy, orthopaedics, analgesics and the correction of any other pathological conditions found in the patients with a view to improving the general health. Specific anti-rheumatic treatments such as vaccines and gold were doubted, rejected or accepted by various observers. Since then steroids have been used with disastrous results, although by now most of their abuses have been mitigated. Anti-inflammatory drugs have been more recently introduced.

Douthwaite [8] summed up the position in 1948 by pointing out that

> Accepted nomenclature connotes a much wider field of disease to
> some than it does to others, causation still remains unsolved and
> treatment is, not surprisingly, in a highly unsatisfactory state.

Over 40 years later neither causation nor treatment has made any
practical progress.

In this scientific era, I believe that investigation of the joints has so far
yielded little of proven value, and while the more recent excursions into
genetics may eventually explain how the pathology develops, they will
not identify the original cause of the pathology.

Let us look first at the classification of the chronic rheumatic diseases
as laid down by The American Rheumatism Association [9] and The
Annual Report of the British Committee on Chronic Rheumatic Disease,
used in all standard books on arthritis. These are very similar and both
deal with the various arthritides and soft tissue pathologies as separate
entities. All standard textbooks follow this plan and thus help to
maintain the concept of the independence of these diseases. The main
classifications are as follows, but it is claimed that there are about 200
different forms of arthritis:

Rheumatoid arthritis
Osteoarthrosis
Spondylitis
Gout
Infective arthritis
Psoriatic arthritis
Hormonal arthritis
Reactive arthritis
Paediatric arthritis
Lupus erythematosus
Polymyalgia rheumatica
Soft tissue disease such as fibrositis

I cannot accept this classification of the chronic rheumatic disease on
the grounds that it is based on an analysis of already-established disease
processes of many years' duration, and overlooks the prediagnostic
clinical evidence which suggests the possibility that they may have a
common origin. It seems to me that different forms of arthritis might be
the end-results of a common systemic disease. These end-results could
be varied by so many intercurrent factors that differences, rather than
similarities, are noted and emphasised in the clinical pictures presented.

Furthermore, segregation of non-articular disease from the arthritides tends to create a mental block about their possible continuity, and thus impedes the concept of a comprehensive pathological process. In view of the failure of this method of analysis to solve the problem of arthritis, a new approach is needed, whereby we seek for the similarities and common factors which can point to a relationship between them. It is the probable unity of these apparently different clinical pictures which makes them more easily comprehensible and thus more available to treatment and prophylaxis.

The concept of this unity is based on the belief engendered by clinical observations that there is a common infective factor in all cases of chronic rheumatic disease. This infection starts as a systematic invasion primarily affecting the connective tissue and is very likely to be viral in nature.

From a study of hundreds of case histories it seems fairly certain that the connective tissue lesions result from an infective process such as upper respiratory tract virus infections and (in children) infectious diseases such as chickenpox and measles. The aching, pain and restriction of movement are caused by the inflammatory involvement of the connective tissue in the related areas, and these are designated rheumatic patches (chapter 4). It is only at a much later period that arthritis develops in the joints related to these patches.

Careful clinical examination will always reveal both conditions when arthritis is the presenting symptom. The soft tissue lesions are always related to the affected joints and their onset can be traced back by detailed knowledge of the history and examination. The lesions may completely subside and leave no ill effects. However, on the other hand, the locally affected areas may persist as rheumatic patches and give rise to stiffness, aching, pain and loss of power or movement.

Repeated attacks may aggravate the already existing areas and also lay down new ones. The disease process then becomes cumulative and the areas longest affected determine the onset of arthritis in the related joint. This may present as rheumatoid arthritis, osteoarthritis, or whatever classification it most nearly resembles. Thus rheumatoid arthritis would present around the second and third decades and osteoarthritis around the sixth and seventh decades.

It is fully realised that all doctors have been taught and trained that arthritis of whatever kind is a disease of the joints and that there are about 200 different types of arthritis. Decisions as to what type of arthritis a particular patient has are made after X-raying the joint and laboratory tests. As a result of this, research has been concentrated mainly on joints although there are now more papers published on the connective tissue—a very welcome sign.

Because of this 'traditional' approach, readers may find it very difficult to adjust their attitudes to a concept of arthritis as only a secondary result of an inflammatory condition of the connective tissues, with the 'rheumatic patch' as the key factor (a full description of the patch is given in chapter 4). Equally unacceptable may be the possible common relationship between a case of rheumatoid arthritis and osteoarthritis of the hip. It is the vital link between the soft tissue disease and the clinically recognisable arthritis which I hope to prove and thus to use to point the way to a better understanding and treatment of the chronic rheumatic diseases.

RHEUMATISM AND ARTHRITIS   (D.J.L.F.)

'Rheumatism' is a non-specific term encompassing all sorts of musculo-skeletal aches and pains. 'Arthritis' is a much more specific term meaning inflammation of a joint. The separate terms 'rheumatoid arthritis' and 'osteoarthritis' carry the implication that the causes of the two types of arthritis are different. Our contention is that the pathologic-al changes in the joint itself, although certainly interesting and very different between osteo- and rheumatoid arthritides, are only of secon-dary importance. The main seat of mischief is not in the joint but in the soft connective tissues associated with the joint and sometimes a considerable distance away from the joint. As evidence for this conten-tion, Bill Fox advances his clinical results: once the relevant rheumatic patches are injected the patient's symptoms become very much better, irrespective of any pathology within the joints. Thus, the pain, stiffness, weakness and often the swelling fade rapidly, frequently within mi-nutes, once the rheumatic patches are injected.

It is therefore necessary to make crystal clear, and constantly to bear in mind while reading this book, the distinction between alleviating the symptoms and alleviating the pathology. We are mainly concerned with the former: so are our patients.

The pathology of the rheumatoid joint, and that of the osteoarthritic joint, have both been classically described [30]. Briefly, in rheumatoid arthritis the first sign of mischief within the joint is oedema of the synovium, followed by precipitation of fibrin at the synovial surface and infiltration by granulocytes. These are followed by variable necrosis of subjacent synovial cells, then reactive hyperplasia of connective tissue cells and formation of new synovial cells. Cartilage is eroded, apparently by the newly formed 'mesenchymal' synovium, which can form itself eventually either into reasonably normal synovium (when the disease is in remission) or into scar tissue (pannus) when it remains active. A puzzling additional feature is the behaviour of the tissues around the joint very early on in the disease process, too early to be the result of the arthritis. Thus, the joint capsule and ligaments stretch, there is atrophy of the muscles, and juxta-articular osteoporosis (thinning of the bone just beneath the joint surface) takes place. Apart from this, rheumatoid arthritis in a joint displays nothing but the typical characteristics of acute inflammation, and tells us nothing about the causal factor(s).

INFLAMMATION

Inflammation is the body's response to an external 'insult'. It can occur anywhere in the body when that part is damaged by infection, trauma, heat, cold or radiation, or toxic chemical exposure. It is quite wrong to think that inflammation is only caused by germs. Inflammation is the body's way of removing the insult (germ, chemical), mopping up and removing the debris of dead cells and damaged tissue, and repairing or at least limiting the damage. When this process is successfully accomplished within a few days we see acute inflammation. When the insult is more persistent, and cannot so easily be removed, we see chronic inflammation. All the microscopy of rheumatoid arthritis tells us is that there must have been an 'insult' of some kind, against which the joint tissues are reacting with acute inflammation. Because in rheumatoid disease the pathology usually progresses to chronic inflammation, we can conclude either (a) that the body is making a terrible mistake or (b) that the insult is an unusually persistent one and refuses to be removed.

If we believe that Mother Nature is usually right, and regard the first explanation as implausible, we then have to ask some very searching questions about the putative insult: what type of material refuses to be removed from the body? We can fairly easily rule out heat, cold, trauma and radiation. That leaves either infection of some kind or toxic chemical exposure, or both. This question is discussed on pp. 59–71.

Where in the body should we look in order to identify the insult? Common sense would suggest that we should look for the cause at the site of inflammation, that is, within the joint. Although infective arthritides certainly exist, they are not rheumatoid disease. Numerous microbiologists have searched diligently over the years for infective agents in rheumatoid synovium and synovial fluid, but with scant and contradictory results [28]. On the other hand, much experimental work in rodents suggests that joint inflammation can be secondary to an insult administered elsewhere in the body.

Adjuvant arthritis, for example, can readily be induced in rats by subcutaneous injection of certain microorganisms. Collagen arthritis can be given to rats and mice by immunising them against type II collagen [27, 40]. These animal models are described in detail on pp. 60–61 but the principle is clear: inflammation of a joint can be induced by injecting an insult substance into the *skin* at some distance away from the affected joint. The same lesson should be learned from reactive arthritis (see later) of humans. To confuse the issue further, the synovial fluid from rheumatoid joints is itself inflammatory when injected into mice [29], from which we may infer that the elusive insult substance(s) might yet be present in the joint cavity.

CHAPTER 3

The Clinical Evidence

A COMPOSITE CLINICAL PICTURE   (W.W.F.)

In order to create a basis of understanding for discussion, I will present a detailed case history of what I consider to be a common and typical case of chronic rheumatic disease in the third and fourth decades. From this picture we may trace the history back to childhood and can also see its continued development into the later decades in older people.

The first outline was based on 111 cases and published in 1950 [3]. It has since been modified and made more precise with the experience of many hundreds of cases since that time. The initial essential conception of unity and infection has been strengthened to a virtual certainty by an initial high success rate in treatment and almost one hundred per cent precision in prognosis.

Not all the signs and symptoms will be found in every case, partly because people vary in their reaction to a disease process, and partly because their memory may not be so reliable, or indeed they may not have been asked the right questions.

Nevertheless, once you have learned to probe the history of each case, enough evidence will be accumulated to substantiate the general outline of the clinical picture presented, and it is from this that I was able to unravel the thread entangled in the agglomeration of different types of arthritis.

Presentation of a Typical Case of Rheumatic Disease

Patient
Married woman. Age 34 years. Occupation: secretary. Two children aged 6 and 8 years. No daily help.

Complaint
Right knee painful and swollen for 2 weeks with aching and discomfort in both legs for 4–5 weeks. Last 2 months had general lack of energy.

11

Depressed and nervy, sleeps badly. Mild sweating on effort and sometimes in bed. Palms of hands damp. Present symptoms first started after a mild sore throat. Many similar attacks during the last 5 years. Attacks getting gradually more prolonged and a little more frequent. During last 12 months had only one period of 4 weeks feeling really well, in June last. Smokes: average. Drinks: very little.

History
Right sciatica 4 years ago.
Lumbago 8 years ago and worse during childbearing period.
Appendicectomy 12 years ago.
Tonsils and adenoids removed 20 years ago.
As a child, frequent sore throats and 'growing pains' in knees.
Menstrual cycle 5–6/30. Dysmenorrhoea and 4 days of premenstrual backache and depression.

Examination
Right knee swollen and painful.
Both ankle joints tender over external lateral ligament.
Marked tenderness on pressure over right lumbar spine.
Skin areas of hyperaesthesia related to nerves arising from lumbar 2, 3, 4.
Throat shows increased deep redness around tonsil beds, fauces and uvula.
Temperature 99 °F. Pulse 98 bpm.

Investigations
Blood count shows relative lymphocytosis. ESR 7.
Electrophoresis normal.
Rheumatoid factor negative.
Temperature chart shows variation of 97–100 °F.

Comment on her Symptoms
The patient's history of sore throats, mild sweating, growing pains, lumbago, depression and tiredness would not have been elicited unless she had been specifically questioned, because most of these symptoms did not make any lasting impression on the patient, who was concerned only with the immediate problem of pain and depression.

The raised temperature was discovered only because the patient was able and asked to take thermometer recordings every morning and evening. It was usually normal in the morning after a night in bed and raised in the afternoon or evening after physical work. Aching and discomfort followed the same pattern, i.e. better with rest and worse with exercise. It is important not to confuse this aching and discomfort with pain and stiffness, which is a later and different aspect of the disease and will be discussed subsequently.

The patient became depressed and nervy because she never felt well and could not cope with her housework and children. As she had nothing to show for her symptoms, until the knee became swollen, she had failed to win the sympathy and understanding of her husband or doctor.

As indicated in her history the general condition improved after a time, but recurred at variable intervals. In her case the remissions became shorter and the exacerbations lasted much longer. It was the swollen knee joint which could be seen that alerted the doctor to the reality of arthritis. The long history of growing pains in the knees, lumbago, sciatica, aching legs and tiredness had not been collated or associated with the possibility of arthritis.

Exacerbation of backache and depression occurring 3–4 days before the onset of menstruation was related to the dysmenorrhea and this will be discussed later.

The mild sweating, aching in limbs, tiredness and raised temperature all suggest an infective process not unlike mild influenza. The almost normal sedimentation rate indicated a non-acute illness and the relative lymphocytosis is a very common finding in virus infections.

Physical Examination
The knee was moderately swollen and extremely tender to touch. Careful and detailed examination indicated that the pain was acutely felt by the patient when the skin and connective tissue were handled as distinct from pressure on to the joint or its movements which were also painful.

There were one or two such patches in the skin and the connective tissue above the joint which were exquisitely tender to pressure or pinching. Over the lumbar spine there was again acute tenderness on slight pressure with a blunt rounded instrument (which I call a seeker) over the intervertebral spaces at the lumbar 2, 3 and 4 levels on the right side. There was also some marked hyperaesthesia along the lateral cutaneous nerve of the thigh and the distribution of lumbar 3 over the buttock.

Examination of the throat showed the tonsillar bed, fauces and uvula to be deeper red than the other mucuous membranes, and a suggestion of oedema of the fauces and the uvula which was curled over towards the right side instead of being central.

When all these symptoms and physical findings are correlated you have a picture of a patient who had repeated attacks of a non-acute infective nature associated with either a mild sore throat or a mild influenza giving rise to sweating, tiredness, aching in the back and limbs and depression. The attacks underwent remission and exacerbation over the years. Later the generalised aching became painful in a more localised area, and finally the swollen and painful knee joint developed.

Note how this patient had pain in her legs as a child, elicited only by questioning. At the onset of menstruation, backache developed during the premenstrual period. By the age of 27 she developed persistent backache, which worsened in the premenstrual period and after pregnancy. This was followed four years later by a more localised pain— sciatica on the right side. This was followed four years later by a still more localised condition—pain and swelling in the right knee.

A consideration of all these facts suggests that the arthritis proper developed after a long period of repeated infective processes which were first generalised, and later became localised in the connective tissue related to the affected joint, and finally the joint itself became swollen and tender.

It must be clearly understood that the apparently facile analysis of this one case was made possible only as a result of painstaking questioning and examination of hundreds of cases from which I was able to construct an intelligible picture of the disease process. This clinical sequence offers reasonable grounds for believing that arthritis might be a localised and end-result of a previous generalised infective condition which established a pathology in the connective tissues related anatomically to the joint. The evidence for this statement will become quite clear as I discuss the detailed findings and treatment in a subsequent chapter.

I know that this sort of clinical picture has not been visualised, say in osteoarthritis of the hip, by either orthopaedic surgeons or rheumatologists, simply because it is first seen by them as a painful walking and weight-bearing problem in a diseased hip joint. The history in all of these types of cases can be traced back for probably 30 years, but the patient is not aware of the sequence and is concerned only with the recent illness. Most of the past is forgotten and can be recalled only if the right questions are asked.

On the other hand, in rheumatoid arthritis a similar sequence is discernible in a very much shorter time. It is as though you have a film which in the one case is slowed down and in the other speeded up. To continue the simile, the film could be speeded up at one stage and slowed down at another. Also, the film at different stages, could be over- or underexposed. With all these combinations, very different impressions can be caused by the same film, and indeed will not even be suspected or recognised as the same film by the majority of observers.

However, from the above information, this case can be recognised as rheumatoid arthritis with a raised ESR, a positive rheumatoid factor, and minimal X-ray joint changes.

COLDS AND SORE THROATS, PHARYNGITIS

When patients are asked about their symptoms they invariably refer to colds, sore throats and pharyngitis as a 'cold'. I believe that doctors accept this generalisation without question, much as I did until detailed analysis of all symptoms associated with rheumatic disease was undertaken. It then became clear that what most patients called a 'cold' was really a mild sore throat or pharyngitis. In fact, it soon became obvious that the patients hardly ever had colds; they were invariably sore throats which preluded an exacerbation in the rheumatic symptoms.

The importance of distinguishing a cold from the other symptoms depends on the understanding we attach to them. A cold is characterised by nasal catarrh and obstruction, sneezing, and generally feeling unwell. The symptoms persist for three or four days when suddenly the patient feels very much better, the catarrh ceases and there are no after-effects.

In clinical terms, this represents an attack by a virus, which has been contained by the body defences and expelled via the catarrhal discharge—it can often be identified in the laboratory. This clinical picture represents a healthy person quickly overcoming an infective agent. In contrast, the sore throat or pharyngitis represents the failure of the body to overcome the virus, which is then able to penetrate the defence mechanisms. It then attacks the connective tissue, giving rise to all the symptoms described in this chapter.

What has proved most interesting is that patients who make good progress will, after a year or two, develop their first real cold since the disease started, which may have been many years before. When this happens, it signifies improved resistance of the patient and improves the prognosis.

It is not inappropriate at this point to refer to my book *Arthritis—Is Your Suffering Really Necessary?* published in 1981 [11]. Its purpose was to educate sufferers about their disease and how to cope with it. In publishing terms, it was a best-seller, being reprinted five times in the first year and then issued in paperback.

The first year brought 1600 letters from readers—'phenomenal' was the remark of the publishers. By 1986, the number of letters had reached over 6000. What is important about these letters is that the content was the same: 'You have described my illness exactly'; 'You have helped me to understand my illness and made it easier to cope'; 'You have removed the guilt feeling I suffered about my tiredness and inability to cope'. All these sufferers were confirming the truth of the clinical story compiled from the interrogation of patients over 17 years.

It is hoped that what the patients have found to be true will encourage the medical profession to accept the reality of the detailed clinical story described in this book. Evidence and further discussion of this problem will be dealt with in the following chapters.

ORIGINS OF RHEUMATOID ARTHRITIS AND PROGRESSION TO OLD AGE

In chapter 2 I presented a typical case of chronic rheumatic disease in a woman aged 34. We should now consider how this kind of case could have developed from childhood and how it might continue through to old age.

There are many children who develop acute pain in an arm or leg or even in the trunk at the ages of 5 to 10. Many are investigated but are hardly ever diagnosed because, with rest, the symptoms soon clear up and a possible rheumatic cause has not been suspected. The episode is forgotten and there may be no recurrence at all, or not for some years.

It must be conceded that most children do not want to be ill and in order to go out and play they will ignore a mild pain or discomfort. In any case, most of them respond to a little rest and an aspirin but in some children the pain and discomfort become more persistent and then a precise diagnosis must be made. I will quote the case of a girl of 9 who developed a recurrent pain in the left mid-abdominal area which was always worse at school. She had been seen by her local GP, who referred her to a consultant and she was investigated in a paediatric department of a teaching hospital. Nothing at all helpful emerged and, on the face of it, it looked as if the child did not like school and this was a good excuse to stay at home, which she frequently did. On examination, I discovered a localised rheumatic patch related to dorsal 11 and 12. After treating this area the pain cleared up and she returned happily to school. The pain was caused by sitting at a desk and seat unit which was too low for her, making her bend forward and thus involving the rheumatic patch.

The reason this is mentioned now is because, clinically, it is exactly the same as all the milder and more transient cases which are forgotten, except that there was no spontaneous recovery in her case.

Once you appreciate this clinical picture of early chronic rheumatic disease, how and where to look for the affected areas, there will be no difficulty in comprehending its rheumatic nature. You will then be in a position to alleviate the symptoms and institute the necessary steps to inhibit its recurrence.

About the age of 9 some children develop 'growing pains' in the legs, which again is the same sort of pathology in a different anatomical area. Detailed inquiry will often establish that the pains are transient and can often be related to an upper respiratory infection such as a cold or sore throat. In the second decade girls tend to get recurrences, with backache as a prominent symptom, associated with the onset of the menstrual cycle, particularly if there is any irregularity or dysmenorrhoea. During this decade the teenagers will still be liable to occasional attacks of aching or discomfort or even pain, with many of the general symptoms already described and practically always identifiable with 'flu-like, upper respiratory or throat symptoms. Again it must be stressed that, just as in children, most teenagers will tolerate some discomfort so as not to interfere with their social activities, and usually an aspirin gives them the relief they need. It is only those youngsters who do not seem able to overcome the disability who visit the doctor, and because of its 'triviality' not many dare to bother the overworked practitioner too often, and so the seeds of future rheumatic disease are sown.

During the second and third decade recurrence or aggravation of the original symptoms can be related not only to the infective factor but also to the condition of work and stress. It is during the childbearing period and the strain of running a household that in many women general aching and vague pain develops into the first frank recognisable signs of more localised pain. These areas of pain may occur in the back and/or a limb. Those in a limb are generally closely related to a larger joint or to a hand or foot. When a swollen joint or joints appear they are designated as early rheumatoid arthritis, osteoarthritis or 'mixed arthritis'. Those, however, which do not develop swollen joints at the time are not recognised as arthritis at all. You will understand that in order to qualify for the tag of arthritis as laid down by the Rheumatic Council, there must be obvious clinical and X-ray evidence of it. In these early cases the disease has not been going long enough to cause degeneration of the bones or cartilage which would show on X-ray, and so 'the patient has not got arthritis'. It is parallel to saying that a patient cannot have pneumonia unless consolidation of the lung is proved by X-ray, or even worse, that a patient cannot be suffering a coronary thrombosis until the electrocardiograph shows it.

About the fourth decade the more generalised aching tends to lessen and is replaced by more precise and localised pain with or without a swollen joint. Stiffness in the morning after lying in bed or during the day after sitting for some time now becomes a definite symptom which, however, passes off fairly quickly on movement. At this stage the patients will not often mention it unless they are specifically asked because it is so transient and is not so important to them as the pains and disability. Later, because of its persistence, it becomes a feature of the illness.

Many of these patients get an acute attack of pain in an arm or leg which will render the limb unusable for a variable period. By this time, most will have developed enough joint disease to have been classified as rheumatoid, mixed, osteoarthritic, spondylitic, or even menopausal arthritis.

In outlining the picture of chronic rheumatism based on this one case, it must be emphasised that at any stage in its history the condition in any given case may come to an end and no further pathology develops, i.e. the patient has developed an immunity to the disease. From this happy state there are, unfortunately, all gradations of the disease varying from long periods of remission lasting many years to the rapidly recurring ones where the disease reaches an advanced state at a much earlier age.

When the disease becomes active, there is a recurrence of generalised aching, transient and indeterminate pains in various areas, and increase of pain in areas previously affected, with some of the general symptoms of tiredness and mild sweating. This sweating and aching is, however, rarer in older patients when stiffness becomes a more marked feature.

One of the most reliable indications of a possible relapse in a patient of any age who has been well for some time is a feeling of tiredness and some depression. When the disease is quiescent the patient suffers only the recurrent depressing repetition of pain and disability in the same areas. In this state they do cope much better with the problem because they feel better in themselves and the 'tablet' in favour with the medical profession at that time relieves the pain or at least ameliorates it.

It is vital to appreciate and recognise these clear periods of remission and relapse in the activity of the disease because treatment must be modified and its value assessed in relation to the actual state of the disease process at any given time.

It is my impression that the success of many forms of treatment and drugs is often wrongly attributed to them because they happen to coincide with a spontaneous period of remission. I am sure that the reader will be satisfied that every precaution has been taken to avoid this trap in the assessment of my own methods of treatment.

ANALYSIS OF CLINICAL FINDINGS

Having outlined a picture of the chronic rheumatic disease which I trust is coherent, the next stage is to analyse the symptoms and physical findings to see whether they substantiate the original conception. The first problem must be the question of pain, and for this investigation osteoarthritis of the hip was chosen [6]. Clinical observations showed that:

1. Pain can be severe with X-ray evidence of minimal arthritis.

2. Pain can be quite mild with X-ray evidence of advanced arthritis.
3. Pain varies in severity and sometimes even disappears for a time during the course of individual cases.
4. In bilateral osteoarthritis, pain is sometimes more severe on the side with X-ray evidence of less arthritis than the other. The converse is also true.
5. The pain may begin or become worse whilst the patient is:
   (a) lying in bed on the affected side
   (b) sitting in a chair
   (c) attempting to move the limb after sitting or lying
   (d) in persistent movement such as walking or climbing stairs.

It would appear logical to deduce from these facts that the arthritis cannot be the primary and only cause of the pain, otherwise the pain should be there almost constantly and certainly made worse by movement or weight bearing. For example, we are all aware of cases where the patients experience pain in starting to walk but with persistence it eases off and they can walk for a short while with less or no pain even though it returns after a while.

Having accepted this conclusion as a basis for further investigation, it followed that some other cause for the pain should be sought. Therefore I analysed the anatomical pain distribution in 14 patients with osteoarthritis of the hip. The commonest and most precise areas were:

1. In the groin.
2. On the outer aspect of the hip joint.
3. Along the outside of the thigh sometimes to the knee or even below.
4. Lumbar backache which was overshadowed by the other pains and only realised by the patient on specific questioning.

Any one or any combination of these pain distributions could occur in individual cases. All the patients showed the same surprise at the questions designed to locate the pain. To them, pain and the problem of weight bearing were the symptoms that mattered, but with proper explanations they very soon learned to differentiate the pain distributions. It was then possible to relate this pain distribution to specific movements of the leg, and to pressures on the back or leg when sitting or lying.

For example, a certain movement or even attempt at this movement would bring on a definite pain location, perhaps in the groin or down the external thigh, or both. This sequence would be repeated at each attempt and was then confirmed by passive movement of the leg which brought on the same pain distribution.

Similarly, pains occurring when lying down, or sitting, can be reproduced by repeating the same postures.

Having ascertained the fairly precise distribution of the pain the next stage was to examine the anatomical areas of the pain. There were three ways of testing for pain in any given area:

1. Pressure.
2. Light touching or scratching.
3. Pinching.

Pressure always caused pain in an affected area. The amount of pressure required to cause pain varied considerably in different areas. This did not help very much except in demonstrating the painful area.

Very light scratching of the skin frequently showed marked sensitivity which could be checked very easily with a non-painful area of skin nearby. Here was undoubtedly a state of hyperaesthesia of the skin which might be caused by a local condition, or referred from any proximal areas to as far back as the lumbar plexus, or both.

I next took a fold of skin with the adherent connective tissue and squeezed it between thumb and finger. Sometimes the pain was much the same as with scratching but in others it was excruciating. In these latter cases I was also conscious of some thickening of the skin fold as if the subcutaneous tissues were swollen, suggesting a localised inflammatory area.

If both these tests caused no pain, deeper pressure was tried. Sometimes this produced the pain and it was not difficult to locate the patch below the subcutaneous connective tissue in the deeper ligamentous tissue, tendons or, possibly, muscle sheath. One or more of these three locations could be found in every case where a limb was examined.

In the spinal area it was sometimes possible to cause pain only with fairly deep pressure, and in these cases the pathological area would probably be in the region of the nerve plexus.

At this point I would like to emphasise the importance of experience in gauging the amount of pressure used in helping to decide the location, and indeed the amount of pain. It is obvious that the harder you press with a blunt instrument, the more painful it can become even in normal tissue.

I can assure you that there is no difficulty at all in the superficial and subcutaneous areas. If you are not heavy handed you will very soon be able to demonstrate the medial and deeper ones. Remember, you have not only the local findings but also the pain distribution to guide you to the right area.

A further interesting observation was that, where the patient could not precisely locate the pain, it always turned out to be a superficial and referred type of pain, whereas, if the area was sharply designated and particularly when caused by lying or sitting, then a localised sub-cutaneous painful thickening could be found.

To summarise these findings, it was now clear that pain can be produced in precise areas by definite movements or pressures. These areas of pain can be located and the pain could be either referred or localised, or both.

How I came to analyse this problem of pain can be seen from my earlier investigation on the lumbar spine which showed exactly the same kinds of painful areas, although, at that time, I had not recognised the differences in location.

At that time I had wrongly assumed these tender areas were all directly related to the lumbar plexus because (a) the area of greatest sensitivity seemed to be caused by pressure between the transverse processes of the lumbar vertebrae down towards the plexus, and (b) the pain seemed to be referred along the superficial nerves arising from the plexus. I decided at that time to inject the lumbar plexus immediately below the tender areas. For this I used a long needle and injected 12 mg of Depo-medrone in 2 ml of 1% procaine. The solution was released along the track of the needle, saving most of it for the deepest, and as I thought, the most painful part. The idea was that the procaine, with its anaesthetic effect, would very soon indicate whether or not the injection had reached the inflamed area by relieving the pain, and that the Depo-medrone would then activate a healing process which might be more prolonged. The immediate results of a series of 14 cases were very encouraging. Patients were able to walk much more easily and with considerably less pain while the local anaesthetic was effective. Improvement was maintained for some days in some cases but others required more frequent injections. Over a period of more than 12 months it was clear that some of the patients had done very well, others still had pain although better, while others seemed to require too frequent treatment to justify the claim that the Depo-medrone was sufficient to exert a general effect. It was this problem which made me wonder why there were these variations in the results. I then recalled that in some patients there seemed to be a disproportionate amount of pain on pushing the needle through the skin and immediately after.

With the newly acquired knowledge of the sensitive areas, all cases under treatment were now examined with this detail in mind. The painful areas in the lumbar region were tested by the methods described.

I very soon discovered that there were subcutaneous areas of tenderness, and some a little deeper, which I now call medial areas. In the earlier cases, these were the areas through which the needle passed and caused marked pain on its way down to deeper tender areas.

Injection of these subcutaneous and medial areas with procaine produced immediate improvement in the symptoms. Pursuing this line of investigation further, I studied the effect of passing the needle slowly through all the tissues from the skin down to the psoas muscle. It became clear that there were areas of great tenderness and others of total insensitivity. The muscle seemed to be pain free and the tender areas were situated in the superficial and deep fascias, as well as in the region of the plexus. The latter would be hardly surprising, excepting that this again varied in adjacent areas in the same patient, just as it did in the superficial areas.

Comparing these findings with the local ones already described, it seemed clear that over the lumbar spine one could have the same superficial condition of skin hyperaesthesia, subcutaneous pain of a localised condition, or pain on deeper pressure caused possibly by a pathological condition involving the lumbar plexus.

As I had now become anxious about the too frequent use of Depo-medrone in the same patient, I finally decided to try a solution of 0.5% sodium salicylate. This was specially prepared for me and I first tried the effect on myself. I injected it slowly, immediately after piercing the skin of the thigh down to the belly of the muscle. It proved absolutely painless and with no after-effects. I then selected three of my patients, explained the experimental nature of the work, and they agreed to have the treatment and to risk the consequences.

Injection of the fluid without a local anaesthetic produced no pain until the needle met a sensitive area and then the fluid caused intense pain, which lasted about 60 seconds. A further observation, noted when the needle met a sensitive area, was that movement of the needle felt exactly like the bowing of a violin string, which gave rise to anything but a musical note from the patient. After the local anaesthetic had deadened the area, you could still feel this sensation of bowing transmitted through the needle and syringe. Once past the sensitive area, the fluid caused no pain at all, exactly as it was in the personal experiment. It now seemed quite clear that the solution caused no pain in normal tissues, but in what appeared to be inflamed areas the pain became intense for about one minute and then subsided, with a concomitant improvement in the patient's symptoms. The same immediate improvement was obtained with procaine alone, although even with the procaine the injection was painful but nothing like to the same extent, until the anaesthetic effect came into being.

Continued repetition of this procedure in over 100 patients confirmed these definite findings:

1. There are sensitive circumscribed areas of acute tenderness in the superficial and deep fascias, which may occur in any part of the body.

2. The superficial areas are easily identifiable by picking up the skin and subcutaneous tissue, and compressing them between the finger and thumb, when they become very painful.
3. The superficial areas cause pain and limitation of movement of the joint related to them.
4. The superficial areas respond immediately to a local injection of procaine and sodium salicylate by first being painful and then becoming pain free, allowing more freedom of movement of the joint.
5. There are also more diffuse areas of pain elicited by scratching or light pinching, but no worse when a fold of skin is squeezed. Injection of these areas with procaine and/or sodium salicylate causes no obvious improvement in either pain or mobility. These areas should be traced back either to the more localised patches already described or to the lumbar spine, where the appropriate pathology would be found.

I had originally thought the pain was caused by an inflammatory condition of the nerves in the lumbar plexus, but these investigations suggested that it was probable that the nerves were secondarily involved in the pathology of the surrounding connective tissue, although they may also be primarily involved. This would explain why the original deep injection with procaine and Depo-medrone did not always produce uniformly good results: it would be successful only in those cases where the main inflammatory area was in the deep fascial layer and from which the leg pain was mainly referred. No further improvement could be obtained until the subcutaneous areas were treated. It seems likely that, if I had realised this at the outset, treatment with Depo-medrone would have been more successful.

At this stage, the result of treatment in every case was exactly the same: pain was abolished or greatly ameliorated and movement of the leg improved.

It was now possible to understand why the pain was sometimes worse when lying on the affected side. It was because there was pressure on one of these localised tender areas in the connective tissues of the thigh. When this had been located and treated, that particular symptom was removed. The same principle applied to a sitting position.

The treatment of these painful areas also diminished or abolished the pain experienced by the patients when they attempted to move the limb, or when actually trying to change position even when not weight bearing. It was this relief from pain which allowed freer movement of the leg and which could be demonstrated by the patient's taking a longer stride than usual, and quite often being able to raise the leg sufficiently to make going upstairs easier, and, perhaps, more importantly, allowing them to dress, i.e. stockings, socks, trousers, with much less trouble.

With all this evidence it cannot be unreasonable to claim that it must be wrong to assume that pain and limitation of movement are due to the arthritis in the joint.

It now seemed appropriate to investigate in detail some of these localised painful patches. My line of investigation was to take biopsies from five patients.

1. Rheumatoid arthritis. F.W. (male) age 53.
   3 years' history of a rapidly developing type with all the joints of both hands affected and supported with splints. Pain was now developing in both knees and feet.
   Biopsy of skin and superficial fascia removed near the lumbar spine.
   Laboratory report: hyaline degeneration of the connective tissue, thickening of the walls of the blood vessels but no active inflammatory reaction.

2. Osteoarthritis. S.F. (male) age 73.
   Recurrent history of rheumatic episodes over 40 years with lately developing osteoarthritis of the spine and hips.
   Biopsy of skin and superficial fascia removed from near the lumbar spine.
   Laboratory report: connective tissue showed hyaline degeneration and the skin showed a mild focal non-specific inflammation.

3. Non-articular rheumatism. H.W. (male) age 47.
   Sweating. Recurrent episodes of pain in various parts of the body with no obvious arthritic development as yet.
   Biopsy of skin and superficial fascia removed from dorsal spine.
   Laboratory report: connective tissue showed hyaline degeneration and the skin showed a mild local non-specific inflammation.

4. E.S. (female) age 63.
   Undecided by two professors whether rheumatoid or osteoarthritis in both hands.
   Biopsy of skin and superficial fascia removed from left upper arm.
   Laboratory report: connective tissue showed hyaline degeneration and the skin showed a mild local non-specific inflammation.

5. Rheumatoid arthritis. R.R. (female) age 42.
   Biopsy of skin and superficial fascia removed from left upper arm.
   Laboratory report: connective tissue showed hyaline degeneration and the skin showed a mild focal non-specific inflammation.

Although the biopsies were not clinically controlled, I suggest that these clinical findings together with the pathological reports constitute a reasonable basis for a better understanding of the rheumatic disease process, and this is an appropriate moment to summarise the postulate, fact, and conclusions so far discussed.

1. All chronic rheumatic disease is initiated by an infective (probably virus) process, e.g. sore throat or influenza.
2. Pain is caused primarily by a localised inflammatory condition of the connective tissue, designated the 'rheumatic patch'.
3. The histology of these patches is substantially the same whether the clinical picture is non-articular arthritis, osteoarthritis, or rheumatoid arthritis. (However, it should be noted that the pathology of the synovium is markedly different.)
4. The clinical picture is the same in non-articular, osteo- and rheumatoid arthritis. The main difference once arthritis has developed is that in rheumatoid arthritis the tender areas are much more widespread. Therefore, more joint symptoms are present, and the development of the disease is more rapid with much shorter periods of remission. It is not too difficult to visualise it as a more virulent form of osteoarthritis.
5. In all cases of chronic rheumatic disease there are variable periods of relapse and remission. The recognition of the state of any particular case is essential. Without this understanding the wrong course of treatment may be initiated, resulting in failure and false conclusions. The worst possible conclusion is to confuse a natural remission with ineffective treatment.
6. The assessment of each case should be made on the clinical facts elicited from the patient and the findings of manual examination. There should be little disagreement that the ESR is not a reliable indication of the state of the disease, while a negative rheumatoid factor merely suggests that the test is not sensitive enough in the early stage of the disease. A positive result may antedate the arthritis or be present at onset but it is true that some patients never develop a positive rheumatoid factor test as they may have 'reactive' arthritis. Almost every case of established rheumatoid arthritis seen by me— many hundreds over the years—gives an early history of being told that there is nothing wrong with them. Blood tests and X-rays were all negative.

CHAPTER 4

The Rheumatic Patch

INTRODUCTION (D.L.J.F.)

Rheumatic patches are nothing new; they have been 'inadvertently discovered by patients, their spouses, therapists, and nonmedical practitioners' [31] but not usually their doctors. The literature on Swedish massage and acupuncture is fully conversant with them, albeit under different names [32, 33].

Travell and Simons, in their monumental scholarly monograph [34], list the following synonyms for the rheumatic patch:

fibrositis
interstitial myofibrositis
muscular rheumatism
Muskelhärten
Muskelschwiele
myalgic spot
myofascial trigger point
myofasciitis
myogelosis
non-articular rheumatism
panniculosis, panniculitis
rheumatic myalgia
rheumatic myopathy
soft-tissue rheumatism
trigger point, trigger area, trigger zone
Valleix points

numerous anatomical pain terms

As is clear from the language employed, there is general agreement that the main seat of mischief is the muscle and the fascia associated with it, including the connective tissue sheets and fibres that lie within muscles separating the individual fascicles (figure 1). Most workers agree that when the lesion lies within the muscle it is not the contractile tissues themselves that are damaged but the interleaving sheets of connective tissue [120–122]. Bill Fox's chief contribution to this literature is to focus attention mainly on the superficial fascia, that area of connective tissue that lies between the skin and underlying muscle. While not seeking to deny that rheumatic patches can often penetrate into and through muscles, he points out that in order to obtain good clinical results it is not necessary to insert the needle any deeper than the skin and just beneath. Travell and Simons [34], by emphasising the therapeutic benefit to be derived from spraying the skin with vapocoolant [34], appear to be implicitly conceding this point, and other authors have published studies of trigger points purely within the skin [35].

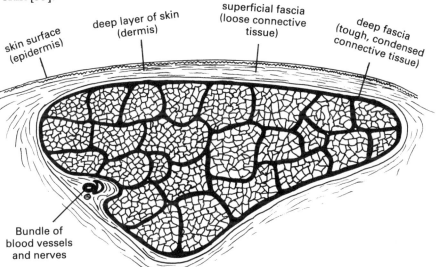

Figure 1 Cross-section through typical muscle, just under the skin. When this muscle contracts, the skin overlying it will bulge. The muscle is entirely invested with, and penetrated by, tough connective tissue. Sheets of connective tissue divide the muscle length-wise into bundles (fascicles). Within each bundle, thinner sheets of connective tissue separate the individual muscle fibres. Within each fibre, microscopically thin sheets of connective tissue subdivide each fibre into fibrils, which are too small to see with the naked eye. These are the actual contractile units of the muscle. The sheets of connective tissue form an interconnected whole, making up a continuous single organ, enveloping and connecting the fibrils, fibres and fascicles so that they can contract semi-independently while remaining closely attached to each other.

There is general agreement that treatment of these patches is reward-ing, whether or not there is also true arthritis present, but there is much disagreement over what the treatment should consist of. Injection of local anaesthetic, normal saline, or even dry needling (acupuncture) all have their exponents, though most concede that any benefit from these procedures is frequently short lived [34, 41, 42]. Ongley *et al.* [36] advocate a solution of glycerol and phenol in dextrose, on the grounds that this solution is highly irritant (i.e. tissue damaging) and would be expected to encourage inflammation (note that rheumatic patches are not inflamed; see p. 31). The 0.5% sodium salicylate solution would appear at first sight to be the direct antithesis of this reasoning, since salicylates are in general anti-inflammatory [39]. We will discuss this in a later section.

We must make quite clear the distinction between a **rheumatic patch**, which is composed of excessive, hard and rather haphazard collagen, and a **rheumatoid nodule**, which is a patch of tissue death and sometimes liquefaction, surrounded by a palisade of inflammatory cells apparently unable to penetrate to the centre of the nodule.

CLINICAL DESCRIPTION OF THE RHEUMATIC PATCH   (W.W.F.)

It is 15 years since *Arthritis and Allied Conditions* [7] was written, and I am satisfied that all the queries and doubts as to the exact cause of pain, aching, and loss of movement have since been resolved by a better understanding of the rheumatic patch.

The rheumatic patch appears to be an inflammatory or post-inflammatory lesion of the superficial connective tissue which becomes adherent to the overlying skin. It can be precisely determined on clinical examination by picking up a fold of skin in the suspected area. When this is rolled between finger and thumb it feels thicker than normal. Light compression becomes unpleasant and is usually described by the patient as pinching. However, a slight increase in pressure becomes painful. Comparison can be made with adjacent areas of skin so that the clinician has no doubt of its reality.

The patch is present in all forms of rheumatoid arthritis, osteoarthritis and non-articular rheumatism; the latter could be more significantly termed pre-arthritic, a term I have adopted. Patches vary from paper thin to 2 mm in thickness with considerable variations in size and shape. These variations are in direct ratio to the length and severity of the clinical picture. For example, in primary lumbago, sciatica or stiff neck there will be one or two patches over the spine related to the area of pain. In osteoarthritis of the hip there are several in the lower dorsal lumbar and iliac areas, whilst in rheumatoid arthritis they are widespread and often coalesce.

The patches can occur anywhere in the connective tissue. No area is immune, except that they rarely seem to appear distal to the wrist and ankle joints. The most common sites are the skin areas over the spinal column, from the base of the occiput to the tip of the coccyx. From these areas, further patches will be found radiating outwards towards the limbs and down to the wrists and ankles.

Histology of the Rheumatic Patch

We now return to the five cases cited above. All five showed hyaline degeneration and lymphocyte infiltration where the connective tissue was adherent to the overlying dermis and were considered to be evidence of non-specific low grade infection.

In 1987, four further biopsies were taken, comprising one case of bilateral osteoarthritis, one case of pre-arthritis, one case of mixed arthritis, and one case of early rheumatoid arthritis (see figure 2).

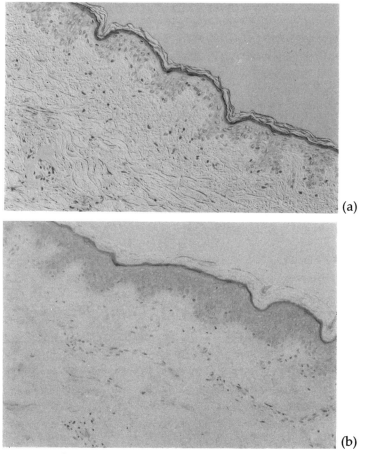

(a)

(b)

Figure 2 *(continued overleaf)*

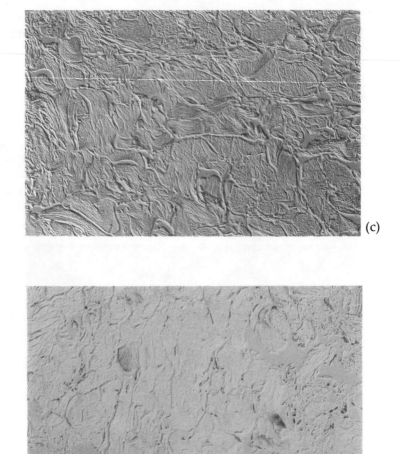

(c)

(d)

Figure 2 (a) Normal epidermis and (b) epidermis overlying rheumatic patch (haematoxylin and eosin; magnification 150×). The normal epidermis is separated from the underlying collagen layer by a layer of looser connective tissue, which is absent in the rheumatic patch. The collagen is more tightly packed in the rheumatic patch and comes right up to the epidermal base. (c) Normal dermal collagen and (d) rheumatic patch dermal collagen (van Giessen stain, Nomarski phase contrast; magnification 500×). In comparison with the normal tissue, rheumatic patch collagen appears more random in its deposition, and contains a sparse but definite infiltrate of lymphocytes (visible at this magnification as dark specks not seen in the normal tissue).

The report of Dr. A. J. Freemont, Senior Lecturer in Osteo-articular Pathology, Department of Rheumatology, University of Manchester, on the sections states that under the light microscope:

All the specimens are much the same.

The biopsies consist of epidermis and underlying dermis. The dermis is uniformly collagenous with irregular thick collagen fibres and a relative paucity of epidermal adnexal structures. The epidermis shows a mild degree of hypergranulosis and hyperkeratosis. There is a scanty lymphocytic infiltrate within the dermis with some cells in a perivascular distribution and some at the dermo-epidermal junction and some lymphocytes within the epidermis itself.

The biopsy sites are not stated but if from back/shoulder/root of neck area the biopsy appearances are within normal limits.

As one of us (D.J.L.F.) commented at the time:

I have examined the sections taken in 1987 and have discussed the appearances at length with Dr. Freemont and with Dr. Hilary Buckley, another histopathologist at the University of Manchester.

The central feature of rheumatic patches can be clearly seen in the photographs: it is a dense patchwork of collagen, with rather fewer of the normal skin appendages (hair follicles, blood vessels etc.) than one would expect. The reader should keep an open mind on the pathologists' mention of perivascular lymphocytic infiltration. Although undoubtedly lymphocytes are there, this is not the dense infiltration of inflammation. Rheumatic patches are neither acutely nor chronically inflamed. The few lymphocytes that we see offer evidence of the immune system's continuing interest in the area, but not of a concerted inflammatory reaction. It should be borne in mind that we have biopsied chronic rheumatic patches, in which any inflammation, if ever there was much, is now long gone and the area is quiescent in terms of active immunological response. We are looking, as it were, at the scar tissue left behind after inflammation, like a deserted battlefield from which the troops have departed. Dr. Freemont notes that dense collagenous deposition of this type is 'normal' in dorsal areas. This does *not* necessarily mean that it is physiological or correct to have it, it could simply be telling us that most humans in our society have dorsal rheumatic patches (as Fox would corroborate).

Dr. Buckley also noted, independently, that in two of these four biopsies the area of collagen deposition was separated from the skin by a thin zone of looser, more 'normal' connective tissue. She wondered whether there was anything different about these two. There was: I had successfully treated these two with dietary manipulation (see pp. 61–3).

I do not believe that one should make judgements on individual biopsies because in a disease which goes on for years there are bound to be differences in histological appearances depending on the length of time they have been there, the amount of stress and strain to which they have been subjected, and not least to the natural recuperative powers of the body.

My own view is that until we are able to take biopsies from people who have absolutely no taint of rheumatic disease in both their clinical histories and clinical examination we can never be sure that any biopsy examined is really normal. Furthermore, in a subsequent chapter I suggest that in order to obtain a true histological picture of a rheumatic patch it should be done as soon as possible after an acute pain develops.

Because the connective tissue envelops the whole of the locomotor system, pathology in one area can and does affect pain and movement in areas distal to it. For example, if you have an early case of rheumatoid arthritis which is affecting mobility and power in the hands and shoulders, injection of the rheumatic patch over the brachial plexus area will produce, within 2–3 minutes, dramatic improvement in the loss of pain, increased power and movement of the arms, wrists and fingers.

Figure 3 shows the dermatomes affected by the cervical and dorsal nerves. This approximately corresponds to the areas affected when a rheumatic patch located over the cervical spine is treated. The only parts of these nerves which could be affected directly by the sodium salicylate injection are branches from the posterior rami supplying the skin of that area. How this comes about is not clear from the present state of our knowledge of the locomotor system, but it will be discussed in a later chapter.

TREATMENT TECHNIQUES

As the disease progresses, more patches are laid down across the shoulders and along the arms. In these circumstances you may not obtain as good an immediate result, because more patches need to be treated, but there should always be enough improvement to satisfy both you and the patient. The technique for treating the patches is as follows.

Select the patch you have decided to treat. Have a 10 ml syringe with an excentric nozzle filled with a 0.5% solution of sodium salicylate and a 40 mm 8/10 needle.

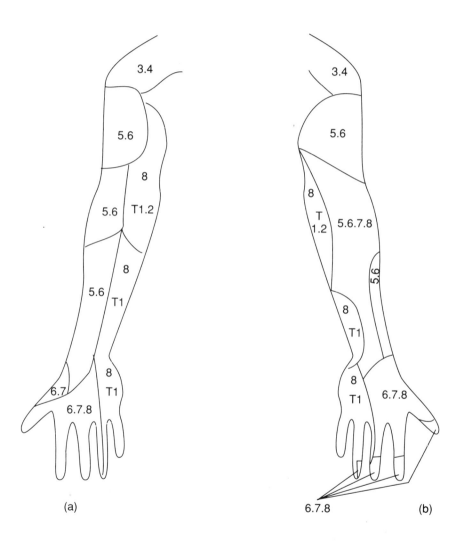

Figure 3 The dermatomes affected by the cervical and dorsal nerves. This approximates to the areas affected when a rheumatic patch located over the cervical spine is treated. (a) Anterior view of the right arm. (b) Posterior view of the right arm.

This should be inserted at the edge of the patch to a depth of 2–3 mm only and the fluid gradually expelled parallel to the skin. As soon as the fluid makes contact with the inflamed area the pain produced is intense but lasts for barely a minute. When the fluid meets that part of the patch which has become adherent to the skin, the pain is rather worse and a peau d'orange effect clearly develops. Once past this area, you may still find sensitive areas and possibly further peau d'orange development (see figure 4).

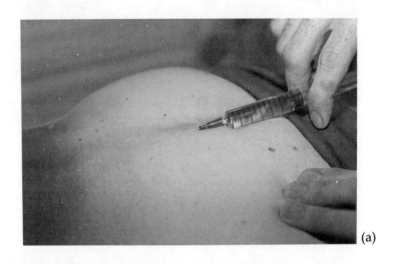

(a)

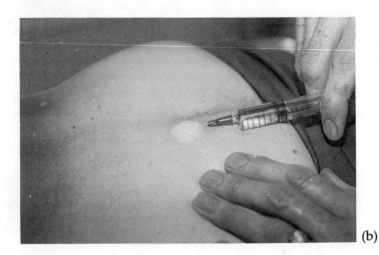

(b)

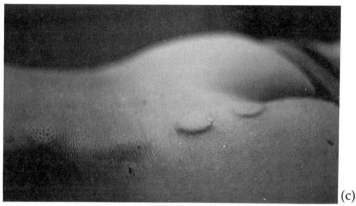

(c)

Figure 4 (a) Operator inserts needle into, and parallel with, the skin, close to the surface so that the outline of the needle can be seen. (b) Injection of 0.5% sodium salicylate to raise a weal. (c) Three treated rheumatic patches, just to the left of the mid-line. The patch on the extreme left shows the 'peau d'orange' effect that tells the operator he has treated the right area.

Complete the treatment with 10–20 ml of sodium salicylate and within 1–2 minutes the patient will demonstrate the improvement by the reduction or loss of pain and increased movement and power of the affected area.

Providing that the injection is done correctly and at the correct site, there are absolutely no exceptions to the immediate clinical improvement.

If the disease process is not in an active state the improvement will be maintained for at least 12 hours, and maybe up to 1 week or more. If the disease is active, then the improvement can disappear in a matter of minutes. This is quite understandable when you realise that the patch injected is a small part of the connective tissue, which is still under bombardment by the inflammatory agent and thus can be quickly re-inflamed. For this reason alone, it is essential to make a clinical assessment of the state of the disease so that you will neither mislead yourself nor disappoint the patient.

During the early years of my researches, the clinical picture which is now so clear was then hazy and indeterminate. Therefore, in order to relate the clinical findings clearly to the possible outcome of the injection, an assessment of the activity of the disease was written into the case history and later compared with the actual result. It was in this way that it became possible to evaluate with confidence the signs and symptoms in relation to the disease activity.

Nowadays the patient is told after consultation and before treatment what the prognosis is likely to be. If there is any doubt, this is also conveyed to the patient, but it is a rare necessity.

The significance of these findings is that local treatment of the rheumatic patches should rarely be done when the disease is in an active state. Where the disease is in remission each treatment will bring a measure of improvement in loss of pain and increased mobility which is sustained for months or years without the use of pain killers or anti-inflammatory drugs. This improvement I believe to be far greater than that achieved by more conventional means. A relapse into activity of the disease process can occur at any time.

Fortunately its onset can be recognised by the patient, because it is preceded by all or some or these symptoms: mild sore throat, generalised aching, lack of energy, depression, and increased pain. It is extremely important that patients should understand this because it mitigates the fear and disappointment which these unexplained relapses engender in so many patients. This aspect will be discussed in more detail under specific treatment.

The distribution and relationship of the patches together with their significance presented a problem which took many years to solve. In the early years patches near the affected joints were treated first, which invariably produced some improvement in loss of pain and increased mobility. At the time it seemed almost miraculous, to both the patient and myself. However, the improvement in many cases was not maintained for more than a few days.

I then moved further away from the joint, proximally, and treated other patches which could be identified. This, in turn, gave rise to further improvement. This process gradually determined that every patch between the affected joint and the spine must be treated to achieve the maximum improvement available. Even a hip joint can be greatly improved but it is a painstaking task because there are so many patches to be done.

With increasing experience, I then began to treat the more proximal patches first and found the results of this manoeuvre to be better and more lasting. What was even more surprising was that the more distal patches, i.e. those nearer to the joint and as yet untreated, became less swollen and less tender. When this process continued, some of these patches did not require any treatment because they virtually disappeared. This favourable outcome occurred mainly in those cases where the disease was not of too long standing, because the longer the history, the more permanent and tougher became the patches.

Inevitably I was driven to detailed examination of the spinal column. It was here that I found, without exception, rheumatic patches along the mid-line from the base of the occiput down to the coccyx.

In all cases with a relatively recent history, and therefore mainly younger people, these patches can be easily identified by the method already described. Injection of the patch showed that the affected area was larger than you would suspect from manual examination, and that if done adequately, the result in loss of pain and increased mobility was quite astonishing.

In older people with a long history it became more difficult to pick up the skin over the spinal column because it had become bound down to the superficial fascia, but the tenderness could still be elicited by attempting compression or by direct pressure. It is in these areas that many of the patches have become thickened and are often so hard that there is great difficulty in forcing the fluid into the patch.

Because of the purely physical problem of injecting the sodium salicylate solution into these hardened areas, it should be realised that a return to such areas is necessary at a later stage in order to complete the healing process and thus to maintain and prolong the improvement initially obtained. Some of the more distal patches can also become as tough as those over the spine. These will also require treatment before the best results are achieved.

These studies over the last eight years leave me in no doubt that the first treatments should be started over the spinal area, and followed where necessary by the more distal patches.

As you can see, the process of treatment has been completely reversed from when I first started to identify the rheumatic patches, with one exception. That was when I first started to treat osteoarthritis of the hip by injecting rheumatic patches which I thought were present in the deep fascia affecting the lumbar plexus. Although there may be some truth in this, it did lead me to the more important discovery of the superficial patches over the spine, and eventually to their primary significance.

When this clinical picture became so clear and unequivocal—more than 80% of all patients treated demonstrated quite remarkable immediate improvement—it brought to mind my studies of osteopathy, one of the subjects I turned to in my early days in general practice because I was so disappointed with the results of allopathic medicine.

I did achieve a few excellent results by manipulation of the spine but the failure rate was high. Was this due to my lack of experience and expertise, or were the ideas propounded by Dr. Still in the last century too all-embracing? What I found so intriguing about his theory that all pain symptoms emanated from the maladjustment of the vertebrae was that he had been so perceptive in realising that not all pain was due to disease of the viscera, the central point of medical teaching and practice.

Because of his undoubted successes where visceral disease was absent, he understandably fell into the trap of believing that all disease was initiated by spinal maladjustment. Remember, the establishment of cause and the diagnosis of most diseases were in their infancies in those days.

From this polarisation of viewpoints, it is now understandable why he was an anathema to orthodox medicine. Over the years, more knowledge in both fields has brought better understanding and tolerance, so that, in the USA, osteopathy is legally recognised as an acceptable form of medical practice. In the UK, although not given the same status as in the USA, it is practised by an increasing number of the medical profession.

However, the facts are still the same; it has no value in treating visceral disease and does not succeed in the large number of cases which I refer to as the undiagnosed masses of patients who fill the GPs' surgeries and hospital outpatients' departments.

I have now found that the most important rheumatic patches are located under the skin immediately over the spinal column. These areas must surely be what Dr. Still found when he examined his patients. One can assume that most of them were middle aged or older so that many of the rheumatic patches would be scarred and inactive, thus causing some maladjustment of the vertebrae (this will be fully discussed in a later chapter).

Manipulation of these areas would restore the normal bone relationship especially at the facets, and no doubt would result in the alleviation of the patients' symptoms. If, however, the disease was active with inflamed rheumatic patches, manipulation would obviously do no good, and persistence would make matters worse—you cannot improve an inflammatory situation by massage or manipulation; it is against the basic orthodox treatment.

I think that this analysis of the problems of osteopathy is correct. Perhaps the evidence you need comes best from osteopaths and other related practitioners.

In 1982 I lectured to the Anglo-European Osteopathic Association at the Royal London Homeopathic Hospital where they were holding their symposium. I demonstrated the diagnosis and treatment on two volunteers; the Secretary of the Association was the first, and the second came from the audience.

Although my remarks made it clear to them why they had so many failures, they showed their appreciation in one of the most remarkable demonstrations of enthusiasm for the truth that I have ever experienced.

Three years ago I taught a doctor of osteopathy in the USA, and his enthusiasm for the understanding of his failure has made him a total convert to my theories and practice.

In 1989, a demonstration on 3 volunteers from an audience of nearly 300 members of the London and Counties Society of Physiologists, whose practice includes manipulation and massage, was overwhelming because of the clear success of the treatment. Since that demonstration, there has been a considerable feed-back from members who are anxious to improve their knowledge and practice.

Analysis of Treatment

— There were 796 patients, 285 males and 511 females.
— Age range 15–92 years, average 54 years.
— 36 were pre-arthritic.
— 204 had rheumatoid arthritis.
— 556 had osteoarthritis.
— All patients having current steroid therapy were excluded.
— Treatment consisted of 20 ml of a 0.5% solution of sodium salicylate injected into rheumatic patches at weekly intervals.
— The number of treatments varied from 2 to 40, giving an average of 16 per annum.
— Response criteria were judged by increased mobility, marked reduction or abolition of pain, discontinuation of non-steroidal anti-inflammatory drugs, analgesics (except for the occasional aspirin tablet), and the cessation of physiotherapy.

Table 1 details the results of treatment in 1982 and 1983.

Table 1 Results of treatment over a two-year period (1982–1983) [12]

		Improved	
	N	4 wks	12 wks
Pre-arthritis	36	36	36 (100%[a])
Rheumatoid arthritis	204	116	152 (75%[a])
Osteoarthritis	556	335	440 (79%[a])
Total	796	507	628 (79%)
Local reaction or pain intolerance	16 (2%)		
No initial improvement	31 (4%)		

[a] Maintained for 1–2 years.

I am fully aware that these figures relating to treatment do not satisfy the rigid standards laid down for double-blind trials. Quite apart from the trials of the effectiveness of the sodium salicylate, this would require that every doctor using the treatment should first be instructed in the recognition and significance of the rheumatic patch because that is basic to the new concept of the chronic rheumatic disease which I am putting forward. For this reason it would seem inappropriate to apply the requirements of a double-blind trial.

However, there are other criteria relevant to this work which are scientifically acceptable. Firstly, the results can be forecast and repeated in any number of patients under controlled conditions with a success rate of 80%. Secondly, the treatment produces the same success rate when done by independent agents who have been trained in the method.

Perhaps the most surprising and quite remarkable support for my claims is contained in a report published in a Bulgarian journal [4] which states that 'after trials in the rheumatology clinic of the Medical Academy in Sofia in 1979 and 1984, treatment of osteoarthrosis showed an 80% improvement rate and is now officially available in every district hospital in Bulgaria.' The treatment consists of the local injection of a sterile solution of sodium salicylate, novocaine and vitamin B. Quite a remarkable coincidence, you might think!

The rheumatic patch is as much a clinical reality as a rash on the skin, a sebaceous or intradermal cyst in the skin or a lipoma under the skin. Its development is closely and clearly related to the detailed clinical history of the chronic rheumatic disease. The chances of a scientific solution of any medical problem must be directly related to how well we understand that problem, and I believe that the rheumatic patch brings us much closer to that understanding and is a vital missing link in our knowledge of the chronic rheumatic disease process.

SODIUM SALICYLATE

You will recall that early research work on arthritis of the hip was carried out with local anaesthetic and Depo-medrone, a drug which I dislike using because its main effect is achieved by suppressing the inflammatory reaction in the tissues, but allowing the disease process to continue — a drug which flatters to deceive both the doctor and the patient. The disappointing and sometimes tragic results of persistence in this form of treatment are all too common.

A decision to replace it with sodium salicylate was made because it is the oldest, most widely used drug in rheumatism and its value in relieving pain is unquestioned. There are no side-effects from the average doses used by millions of people, whilst those that do occur with increased dosages are very well known and reversible (except in those with fatal gastrointestinal haemorrhage).

It seemed quite reasonable to me that, if sodium salicylate could give so much relief when taken orally, injecting an isotonic solution of it directly into a localised rheumatic patch should achieve a similar result with a fraction of the oral dose, and this proved to be correct. 20 ml of sodium salicylate solution contains 100 mg. That is all that is given in one week. Compare that with a minimum oral amount of 300 mg three times a day: 6300 mg orally compared with 100 mg hypodermically—not much chance of any side-effects or complications.

In spite of the fact that salicylates and aspirin have been used for so long, we still do not know precisely how they exert their effect. They are simply classified as anti-inflammatory, and they are known to have profound effects on leukotrienes and prostaglandins.

Dr. Albert Courts, a researcher interested in connective tissue and co-author of a book entitled *Practical Analytical Methods for Connective Tissue Proteins* [13] suggests that, in physicochemical terms, sodium salicylate is a powerful hydrogen-bond breaker. That is, it denatures most proteins very rapidly in the same way that high temperature does more slowly. The reaction of sodium salicylate against normal collagen is to dissolve 1–2% and to cause the fibres to shrink but with most abnormal collagens it did so in far higher proportions. It therefore seems possible that injection of sodium salicylate into the rheumatic patch would help to dissolve away the degenerate connective tissue and possibly denature the virus if present. This should go some way towards an explanation of the beneficial results achieved by injection of the rheumatic patches.

How Does Sodium Salicylate Work?   (D.L.J.F.)

Of all the aspects of this method, the efficacy of sodium salicylate is at first sight the most enigmatic. The early reasoning (p. 40) was that salicylates are known to be anti-inflammatory and effective in rheumatism [39], so why not therefore introduce the drug directly into the lesions that cause the trouble, instead of flooding the whole body and risking systemic side-effects? In that way, it should be possible to achieve therapeutic levels within the lesions with minimal leakage into the rest of the body. However, rheumatic patches are not inflamed (although the histology suggests they once were). Their fundamental abnormality is an excessive and rather random deposition of collagen. This absence of actual inflammation is striking, and leads some to speculate that, if one could only induce inflammation in the lesions, they might resolve. Hence the use by Ongley *et al.* [36] of a strongly pro-inflammatory solution of phenol, noted above, which does in fact induce some therapeutic benefit. So why should an *anti-inflammatory* agent be helpful?

The answer, if there be one, appears to come from the technology of the tanning and glue-making industry, which has amassed a good deal of scientific lore about animal hides and their interactions with various chemical agents [51]. Salicylates are far more than drugs. They have multiple chemical actions that pharmacologists appear not to have noticed. Among these is their chelating ability, that is to say, they mop up and absorb metal ions (cations) and make them unavailable to body tissues [52].

Connective tissue is made up of collagen and elastin fibrils, embedded within and attached to an interfibrillar matrix composed of glycosaminoglycans (GAGs) (see pp. 91 and 93–94), and these attract small cations (positive metal ions) because of their sulphate groups. The cations, in turn, create an osmotic force which attracts and holds water in the tissue, so that it cannot flow (the Donnan effect). Introduce a chelator into such a tissue, so that the ions are made unavailable, and the water should now be able to flow naturally away. Fox has indeed observed this phenomenon on many occasions.

The other main effect of chelators is to uncouple the chemical linkages between the collagen and the GAG matrix [52]. The effect on the physical structure would be profound. It would be as if, in a piece of fibreglass, the glass fibres had all become slippery within the plastic, and could slide freely around. A similar picture is all too familiar in deteriorating reinforced concrete: when the steel bars become loosened within the concrete because of rust, the concrete becomes weak and the building collapses. (After the injection of salicylate into a rheumatic patch the effect can be felt by the palpating fingers within minutes—the stiffness melts away, leaving flexible tissue.)

If this be the true explanation of the salicylate phenomenon, we should find that an even more effective solution to use would be EDTA [52], since this is a stronger and faster chelator.

A further possible explanation (and one preferred by Dr. Courts (see p. 41), for the action of salicylate is its efficacy at breaking hydrogen bonds. Collagen molecules maintain their structure by peptide bonds, which hold the amino acids together in chains, and hydrogen bonds which link adjacent chains together. Although sodium salicylate can uncouple the latter type of bond [53, 54], it does so only at concentrations rather too high (e.g. 32% w/v) to be entirely relevant to the 0.5% solution favoured by Fox. The other objection to this interpretation is that one would have to stipulate some other mechanism, acting at the same time, to uncouple the peptide bonds, unless these were already damaged or incomplete. Perhaps the haphazard collagen in rheumatic patches is incomplete in this way, but we are now in the realm of pure speculation.

LOCAL ANAESTHESIA OF RHEUMATIC PATCHES   (W.W.F.)

In the technique of treatment, injection of sodium salicylate solution only was described. However, during the research period, procaine 0.5% was used initially, because the relief afforded by anaesthetising the inflamed patch gave reassuring evidence that the right area was being treated. The patch could then be infiltrated, painlessly, with the sodium salicylate.

The problem which this method presented was that the operator could never be sure that all the inflamed area had been treated because there was no pain to guide him. The initial injection of the local anaesthetic was quite painful, although perhaps not as severe as the initial injection of the sodium salicylate.

The problem was discussed with the patients. The majority decided that they would stand the pain of the sodium salicylate without using local anaesthetic first, as this shortened the treatment time—an important factor when the tension and strain of the treatment were both mental and physical, and also the treatment was more thorough. Those who preferred the local anaesthetic first accepted its shortcomings, and were able to continue treatment quite happily. Every patient is offered the alternatives and this appears to work very well.

It must be admitted that the original fear of not covering all the inflamed area is minimal because experience and the sense of touch through the needle and syringe constitute a very reliable guide in discerning the difference between normal and inflamed tissues.

However, it seems to me that the use of procaine does minimise the full effect of the sodium salicylate. The effectiveness and duration of improvement are frequently less in those patients electing to have the local anaesthetic. This means that they need to have more treatments to achieve the same result. That is why not more than 1 in 10—usually the teenagers—prefer the procaine.

CHAPTER 5

Causes of Chronic Arthritis and its Treatment

INTRODUCTION   (W.W.F.)

The previous chapter detailed the treatment when the disease is in remission. It is quite simply the local treatment of a localised disease process.

When the disease is active the inflammatory process affecting the connective tissue spreads along that tissue, giving rise to further patches and sometimes reactivating older dormant ones, including those that have previously been successfully treated. In these circumstances, it is essential that all forms of treatment available to combat the infection are given priority over local injections. In practice, the principle of contain-

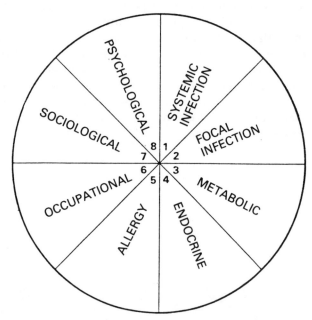

Figure 5 Factors which have a bearing, or are believed to have a bearing, on the disease.

ing the generalised disease process is adopted in all cases in the hope of minimising the chances of recurrence. The strategy employed must be based on every scrap of knowledge we have about the disease, and all the factors which can affect it. Figure 5 covers all the known aspects which have, or are thought to have, some bearing on the disease.

Let us deal with each one in numerical order.

SYSTEMIC INFECTION

Over 50 years ago the possibility of an infective theory was explored, and many organisms were thought to be implicated. It is not necessary to give the details of all the efforts made to produce vaccines, in both this country and the United States, in attempts to combat the disease. None was successful although Warter *et al.* [14] claimed a fairly high degree of success with their combined antigen. As far as I am aware it is no longer in use.

Because the vaccines failed, the infective theory fell into disfavour and was neglected. In my view, this was an error of judgement because, at that time, all that had failed was an orthodox approach to infection, which consisted of immunising the patient with graduated doses of the suspected organisms. It meant simply that we had not yet identified the real pathogen. I was not prepared to reject all the clinical evidence of infection without further effort.

There is no doubt at all in my mind that the detailed clinical study of the case of rheumatoid arthritis described earlier predicates an infective process caused by an external agent, probably viral in nature.

If you have appreciated and accepted the evidence of the vital role which the rheumatic patch plays in the development of arthritis, then you will understand why so much persistent research into the joints has failed to produce any hard evidence of an infective agent. In all probability, that is the reason why a significant number of rheumatologists still have their doubts about the infective theory of this disease.

To increase the chances of isolating the virus, research should be guided by a consideration of the full clinical story. This quite clearly indicates that the onset in very early cases (not recognised as rheumatoid arthritis) and relapses in cases of rheumatoid arthritis are preceded by symptoms suggestive of an infection. These are as follows: mild sore throat (as distinct from acute tonsillitis); upper respiratory symptoms; generalised aches as in influenza; intense tiredness; slight rise in temperature equal to 0.5–1 °F; feeling of malaise and depression; and soon after increase in pain in old areas plus the experience of pain in an entirely new area. In a small number of rheumatoid cases, I have noted the appearance of herpetic spots, looking exactly like chickenpox.

In 1981 Dr. D. A. J. Tyrrell, then Director of the MRC Common Cold Unit in Salisbury, was at the Clinical Research Centre at Northwick Park, London. He had taken some interest in my work and undertook an experiment on the rheumatic patch. This was unfortunately limited owing to expense and other laboratory commitments. Although the culture of a virus was abortive, he felt that the clinical details of upper respiratory symptoms in relation to relapse in rheumatoid arthritis were worth pursuing.

He accordingly arranged for a clinical investigation at Northwick Park, which was published in 1983 [15]. It was set up for 18 children with Still's disease and 25 controls over a period of 1 year. One of the objectives was to document their colds and also the state of their arthritis. He wrote to me as follows:

> The results are probably most clear cut on the clinical side in that there was a statistically significant relationship between the occurrence of an upper respiratory tract infection and a relapse. The second question, of course, was the nature of the upper respiratory infection, and here we were only partly successful, as anticipated. We were able to show that rhinoviruses and streptococci were present in certain colds which preceded the disease. Overall, the number of colds experienced was less than those anticipated but the explanation for this is uncertain.
>
> I wonder whether it would not be a good idea to follow-up your hypothesis by looking for a similar relationship in patients with early rheumatoid arthritis or those who are having a recurrent relapse course. If such a clinical relationship were found then it might be worthwhile looking for viruses specifically. In the case of the Still's Disease I suspect that the abnormality will reside not in the infectious agent but in the type of immune response which is made.

I have already described just these symptoms plus many others heralding a relapse in rheumatoid arthritis, and indeed all those young patients who have all the symptoms and who subsequently develop recognisable rheumatoid arthritis in the second and third decades. Of course, he quite rightly would want to set up similar trials on rheumatoid patients. Unfortunately, Dr. Tyrrell's other commitments supervened, and further work was suspended. To follow up these results, I would like to see a scientific investigation of the throat infection undertaken and a biopsy of a new rheumatic patch which is located precisely in the area of increased pain. The investigation of the herpetic spots could prove very interesting indeed. As we are aware that viruses, like Samson, are quickly destroyed or disappear in the disasters they cause, it is essential that such an investigation is instituted at the earliest possible moment, which means there must be an emergency routine available for the patients under surveillance. This would require the availability of the resources of a hospital unit.

Corynebacteria

Corynebacteria are common bacteria of human orifices without a clear function. I noticed in a series of over 400 throat swab reports of rheumatic cases attending the Charterhouse Rheumatism Clinic that there was a fairly monotonous repetition of six common organisms, all of which had been used in vaccines, without success. However, there was a complete absence of Corynebacteria in all of these reports. I decided to grow throat cultures of all the rheumatic cases under my care with a request to make certain of the presence or absence of Corynebacteria [3]. Fifty-five cases were cultured: Corynebacteria were absent in 47 and present in only 8 cases.

For the purpose of comparison the throats of 50 normal healthy boys attending Highgate School, London, were investigated. They constituted two biology forms and were in daily contact with each other. Their average age was 14½ years. A questionnaire was given to each boy and a verbal explanation of the meaning of the terms used. A copy of the questionnaire is given in figure 6.

Name	*Age* ....
Have you ever suffered from: —	
'Growing pains'	
Cramp in arms or legs	
Rheumatism	
Sore throats	

Figure 6 Questionnaire presented to pupils at Highgate School, London. (It should be mentioned at this point that cramp in the legs and feet, especially at night, is a frequent and persistent symptom in rheumatism. Because it readily responds to the rheumatic treatment described later, it is no longer a problem and is not specifically detailed in the case notes.)

Technique Used

All throats were swabbed at the same time with sterile swabs and these were inoculated on blood agar and cultured for 30 hours at 37 °C. The plates were read under a magnifying glass and doubtful colonies were picked off, stained and examined under oil immersion. Out of 50 throats, 23 grew Corynebacteria. Of the responses to the 50 question-naires, 17 had no symptoms of rheumatism, giving negative answers to all questions, and 7 had marked symptoms of rheumatism, giving positive answers to all questions. 12 of the 17 with no symptoms showed positive Corynebacteria (70%) and 6 of the 7 with all symptoms showed negative Corynebacteria (85%).

This evidence, which is statistically significant ($\chi^2 = 6.52$, $p < 0.01$), indicates that Corynebacteria are more likely to be absent in a rheumatic individual than in a non-rheumatic one. In what way can this be interpreted? Have the Corynebacteria some beneficial effect on their host directly, by elaborating some substance useful to mankind, or indirectly, by acting as a barrier to other bacteria or viruses? A search of the literature for the past 25 years provides evidence only that the Corynebacteria are non-pathogenic to man, that they occur in question-able circumstances as possible involutionary forms and, in one case, as exhibiting an inhibitory influence on avian tuberculosis.

It is fair to draw attention to the fact that all the investigations started with the idea that the Corynebacteria might be pathogenic and it would be most unlikely that evidence suggesting a beneficial effect would have been noted. These results indicated that the Corynebacteria were harmless to mankind, and that they occurred significantly less frequent-ly in rheumatic people than in those free from symptoms.

It seemed not unreasonable to assume that they must have some function. If they were not pathogenic invaders, then they could be normal commensals and perform some useful service for their host, in much the same way as bacteria in the bowel help in the elaboration of vitamin K. For this reason I had a vaccine prepared which has been used ever since. The original report [3] gives all the detail justifying its use and can be referred to if desired. The vaccine consists of: C. *hoffmani* and C. *xerosis* at a combined concentration of 10^9/ml. As a first dose 0.1 ml is almost standard. Occasionally, 0.2 or 0.3 ml may be required and only exceptionally can a patient not accept it because of severe general reaction.

The overall results in 111 cases seemed to be very favourable and I have continued to use it ever since. Obviously its use is empirical, and as there is no exact explanation of how it works I hoped it might introduce into the body some beneficial substance from the Corynebacteria. From a medical point of view this is certainly no worse than using the multiplicity of anti-rheumatic drugs whose action is not understood.

There is now a considerable literature on the Corynebacteria and their anti-viral properties, which appear to be quite remarkable. Werner [16], in a scientific article on immunopotentiating substances with anti-viral activity, gives his own results, and refers to experiments by other scientists, which demonstrate the remarkable power of Corynebacteria to protect mice from virus infection which would normally kill them or render them extremely ill. He suggests that its action may be due to the stimulation of NK cells, probably mediated in part through the production of interferon, and possibly also stimulation of macrophage production. His paper concludes:

> In spite of the impressive experimental evidence in favor of an antiviral activity of *Corynebacterium parvum*, but possibly because of the known complexity of its activity mechanisms and of its side-effects, it does not appear that clinical studies have been performed to demonstrate a beneficial effect of this agent in viral illnesses of humans.

Alas for this poor author who still has so many problems in getting his messages across.

Diphtheroids   (D.L.J.F.)

Of the various bacteria within the genus *Corynebacterium*, most are harmless. Many live as commensals in the normal human throat. One of the species within this genus, *Corynebacterium diphtheriae*, occasionally itself becomes infected by a virus (bacteriophage), and when this happens the virus subverts the bacterium's metabolism to produce a protein which is highly toxic to humans, the diphtheria toxin. Virus-infected *C. diphtheriae*, then, when it goes on to colonise a human throat (or skin) causes the disease diphtheria. It is not the infection that causes damage so much as the intoxication by diphtheria toxin. Corynebacteria in general, apart from this one instance in which they can be converted into pathogens, are harmless and indeed beneficial organisms which serve the function of general non-specific immunostimulators. Because non-pathogenic Corynebacteria look rather similar to *C. diphtheriae* under the microscope, and because their colonies on agar are somewhat similar also, they are loosely termed, in microbiologist's shorthand, 'diphtheroids'.

   Corynebacterium parvum, one of the commonest diphtheroids, has been exploited by immunologists for many years as an adjuvant, that is, it increases the antigenicity of other 'foreign' (non-self) substances. If we wish to produce a good quality antiserum in (say) a horse, against a dangerous bacterial toxin, it is a good idea to inject that toxin together with a dose of *C. parvum* [43]. *Corynebacterium granulosum*, another diphtheroid, has been extensively studied in relation to experimental cancer in laboratory rats, in which state (as in most cancers) the reticuloendothelial system is generally suppressed. *C. granulosum*, and a fraction derived from it called the P40 fraction, can restore several macrophage functions to normal, such as the chemotactic and phagocytic capacities, as well as the ability to withstand infection by herpes virus 1 and *Toxoplasma gondii*. Tumour growth is also inhibited [44, 45].

Bacteria which live harmlessly in the human body are generally termed **commensals**, that is, they 'share the same table' with us in apparent harmony, doing us no harm and deriving no harm from us. In fact, that apparent state of peacefulness is misleading: many of our 'commensals' are actually potential pathogens, and given their chance (if the host's immune mechanisms are damaged by some other, more dangerous infection) they will swarm into the tissues and cause havoc in their own right. These are then termed **opportunistic pathogens**. However, is there another side of the coin? Some indwelling bacteria, we know, are actually beneficial to the host, for example those in the large intestine that produce vitamin K and sometimes vitamin B_{12} on our behalf.

We have already noted a strange thing in rheumatic patients—the unexpected absence of normally 'commensal' diphtheroids from the throats. Could they be, as it were, 'opportunistic symbionts'—that is, given the opportunity would they invade the throat and there cause benefit? The experiment was easy enough to perform. At first Dr. Fox tried spraying the fauces with living diphtheroids, but they did not survive or set up successful colonies. Instead, Fox injected the organisms. (The absence of diphtheroids from the throat, given the normal ubiquity of these organisms, is evidence of some factor in the throats of rheumatic sufferers that actively inhibits their presence. Spraying the fauces would not have been expected to set up lasting colonies.) The organisms were killed before administration, no doubt on general considerations of safety. As we have seen from the animal experiments noted above, the immunostimulating properties of the diphtheroids do not need life in the bacteria: the effect is still there in non-living bacterial fractions.

Influenza Vaccine   (W.W.F.)

There can be little doubt that some of the influenza viruses give rise to rheumatic symptoms. It has been pointed out that, in the detailed clinical case notes of rheumatoid arthritis and in pre-arthritic cases, sore throats or influenza-like symptoms are a regular feature, while many cases can relate the onset of rheumatic symptoms with an attack of influenza. For this reason, all rheumatic cases are advised to have the vaccine every six months and in severe cases as often as every three months.

When this regimen was first introduced some 25 years ago, it became obvious that the standard dose of influenza vaccine was too severe for many of the patients—they became quite ill and the rheumatic symptoms were exacerbated, albeit temporarily. For this reason, patients are given only one-half of the standard dose initially. This immediately disposes of all the severe reactions. It is then followed by a full dose two weeks later. Providing that the dose is continued at least six-monthly, there is no need to return to the half-dose. Where patients are on regular doses of Corynebacteria vaccine, these should be suspended for one week before and one week after the influenza vaccine.

The different ways in which these two methods achieve their objectives suggests that this precaution is wise; simultaneous injections may nullify each other. In practice, the influenza vaccine should be the first line of attack where the clinical picture indicates active disease.

OCCUPATIONAL FACTORS

The problem of the strain of work and travelling is too obvious to need much discussion. The workload applies with equal force to the mother at home with its endless demands on her limited health. It is unfair to expect any treatment to be really successful unless the body is given adequate rest during the active stages of the illness.

SOCIOLOGICAL FACTORS

Here again the problems of damp and bad housing, unhappy household and financial strain do not require anything more than a mere statement of fact to be considered in the pattern of treatment if it is to be successful.

PSYCHOLOGICAL FACTORS

The psychological factor has two important aspects. Firstly, rheumatism may occur in an individual who is primarily disturbed psychologically by other causes, either endogenous or induced by unhappy or misguided family problems. It is important to appreciate this type, because the rheumatic condition may be very minor and merely used as a means of obtaining sympathy. This is very rare in a rheumatic practice, and should present no real problem in diagnosis and assessment. The genuine rheumatic case with an anxiety overlay is very real, and the anxiety stems from a failure to diagnose the condition in its early stages (tiredness, aching, depression and inability to cope with physical demands at school, home or work). Many such patients discover the relief that aspirin and allied compounds give them for a time, but as the illness drags on the depression becomes a major symptom, and tranquillisers are introduced by the doctor to lull the symptoms which have not been understood.

This statement is not an exaggeration, because it is a very common experience in the cases coming under my care. There is a further aspect of the anxiety felt by many patients who see no real progress in their own cases and get depressed at seeing so many older cases, whom they meet in hospital waiting rooms, continuing to deteriorate in spite of treatment.

In 1975 there was a report by Dr. W. A. R. Thomson in the *Daily Telegraph* about some doctors in Ipswich who laudably had eradicated the prescribing of barbiturates from their practice. Writing the article, Dr. Thomson says 'Patients complaining of backache, stiff neck and the like, walk out of their doctors' surgeries with a prescription for the latest tranquillisers.' As backache and stiff neck are very common symptoms of early chronic rheumatoid disease, this statement confirms my view of the general practitioner's failure to understand the significance of the symptoms. Thus they prescribe not only useless and expensive drugs but also potentially harmful ones.

FOCAL INFECTION

This used to be a popular but misguided conception many years ago and was responsible for the wholesale removal of millions of teeth and thousands of appendices and tonsils. There are, however, occasional cases where a septic tooth or tonsil can be justly implicated and its removal may greatly benefit the patient.

METABOLIC DISORDERS AND DIET

The importance of calories and fats in the diet is being constantly overstressed, mainly by the media and the multiplicity of diet experts. Where patients are grossly overweight—very rare in rheumatoid arthritis, except when on steroids—it could be of marginal advantage to diet and it will certainly not affect the course of the disease.

Overeating and overdrinking are the main reasons why people get fatter, whether they have got arthritis or not. Sadly, where arthritis has forced patients to lead a confined and sedentary life, boredom will tend to encourage them to drink or eat more.

The allergic factor is dealt with below.

ENDOCRINE DISORDERS

Ovarian deficiency is the commonest relevant endocrine disorder and it is easily diagnosed by the menstrual history. It may take the form of irregular or painful periods, with 2–5 days of premenstrual depression and backache. The backache is most likely to be an exacerbation of a rheumatic condition which, so far, may not have been bad enough for the patient to seek advice and will certainly not be diagnosed as such. The symptoms subside with the onset of menstruation and are forgotten about, in mild cases, until the next cycle. Even where a doctor has been consulted, medication with analgesics is the usual story. In established cases of arthritis the symptoms are always worse in this premenstrual phase. It is surprising how the patients themselves do not realise it until it has been pointed out to them. It is interesting to note that all the patients who get depression and aching at this time show an increase in weight which decreases after menstruation starts. This is due to fluid retention and can be proved by giving a diuretic which helps to abate the symptoms with the fluid loss. It is not recommended as a standard form of treatment, but merely as an expedient in a temporary situation.

The treatment I use is to inject progesterone in the second half of the cycle: 25 mg on the 15th day; 50 mg on the 22nd day, and the dose adjusted according to the response. In all these cases, the premenstrual syndrome will be greatly improved: the increase in weight, i.e. fluid retention, does not occur, the menstrual periods are normalised, and the rheumatic condition becomes at its least less severe. Nowadays oral progesterone such as Duphaston can be equally effective.

In the fifth and sixth decades the onset of the climacteric brings on similar problems. It is because of this endocrine disturbance that many patients become much worse than they have ever been. Here we see an example of the classification system—it is called menopausal arthritis, and it has been slowly developing for at least 20 years! The treatment in these cases is the cautious use of ethinyl oestradiol to mitigate the endocrine disturbance, always bearing in mind that the menopause is a natural development and should be treated as such. In principle, it would seem wrong to interfere with natural development or regression unless there is good evidence that it is abnormal.

In women, whether married or not, who have lived a fairly celibate existence and where depression is a marked symptom, the injection of small regular doses of testosterone, 25–50 mg monthly, often has a remarkably beneficial effect.

Hypothyroidism is not as rare as may be imagined, and its diagnosis and treatment can be very rewarding in terms of both weight loss and general improvement in the patient's condition. As a rough guide in spotting this condition, increase in weight and a persistently slow pulse should help.

Hyperthyroidism is much rarer and the diagnosis should be established without any doubt at all before any treatment is contemplated.

Diabetes must obviously be properly controlled before there is any hope of treating the arthritis.

ALLERGY

In recent years there has been a realisation that allergy plays a role in rheumatoid arthritis; whether in the chorus or as a star is yet to be determined. As you would expect, all the evidence is based on scientific investigation. One of the first papers was published in 1969 by Broder *et al.* [10], and describes an apparent immune complex in the serum of many patients with rheumatoid arthritis that causes the release of histamine from isolated perfused guinea-pig lung.

This paper is quoted because it demonstrates that allergy in rheumatoid arthritis was discovered almost by accident during laboratory experiments (although it had been suspected for some time). However, the full clinical story of rheumatoid arthritis, as recorded in my case notes, contained clear clinical evidence of allergic reaction in most of the patients. The commonest allergic reactions are as follows: mild localised dermatitis, mostly on the hands; symptoms of mild hay fever; subcutaneous itching, particularly when warm in bed; mild urticaria; and a dislike or intolerance of certain foods. Relevant to these are two cases of rheumatoid arthritis who also suffered from asthma. In both cases, when the disease improved, the asthma worsened and vice versa. In those early days, some of the patients were tested for allergies, but the results were so variable that no great reliance could be placed on them.

These same difficulties are present today, particularly where food is concerned. Because of these problems, I decided to use an antihistamine, initially promethazine hydrochlorate 10 mg t.d.s. The dose proved to be far too strong, causing dryness of the mouth, inability to focus the eyes, and sleepiness. Adjustments were made and a final plan was one tablet taken before going to bed at night. The sleepiness was a real bonus. Most patients slept much better. 'More restful' was the usual response. The dryness cleared by the time breakfast was taken whilst the focusing of the eyes became normal by mid-day. It did cause slight problems in reading the morning papers. The allergies were less troublesome, which added to the well-being of the patient.

Zuraw *et al.* [17] detail the isolation of the IgE factor in rheumatoid arthritis and asthma. I met him when lecturing at Scripps Research Center in La Jolla, California, and he confirmed that the type of antihistamine used in my treatment of rheumatoid arthritis was likely to be the most beneficial.

In my view, allergy does not play a star role in the causation of rheumatoid arthritis because relapses in the disease occur while antihistamine is being taken. Equally, remissions occur in patients whose allergies remain untreated. It is certainly in the chorus and may have a starlet role in some instances. One other symptom which is probably allergic in origin is the swelling of the feet in hot weather. This is probably akin to the turgescence of the bronchi in asthma. Both these conditions can be favourably influenced by the addition of 15–30 mg of ephedrine once daily. Allergy and immunology will be discussed in more detail in chapter 6.

In considering the eight factors in causation, and therefore in treatment, infection is considered as the primary and consistent one. All the other factors are variables and their relative importance can be represented by an increase or decrease in the segment sizes in figure 5 relative to each other. For example, 'endocrine' would occupy most of the space in a case of diabetes, whereas 'allergy' would take a major portion in a case of asthma or dermatitis. The whole plan of treatment for each case can thus be mapped out with special consideration for the factors which emerge as important.

SUMMARY

A summary of the basic treatment used is as follows.

1. Stimulation of the immune system by the use of influenza vaccine and Corynebacteria.
2. Rest when the disease is active with a limited use of aspirin. Because

the disease primarily attacks the connective tissue, you will understand that, particularly in the active stages, movements will tend to spread the inflammation along this tissue. For this reason, rest must be an urgent requirement. This includes the cessation of all massage, manipulation and exercises.

I realise that this is contrary to the popular theory that exercise is important to prevent joint contraction. This theory is well practised and supported in the management of bone and joint injuries, where the injury site is protected by plaster splinting. If this basic principle is applied to rheumatic disease, then you will better understand why the rheumatic patch must be protected from massage or exercise until it has been healed. Only after this stage should the need for physiotherapy be assessed.

3. A small dose of antihistamine at night.
4. Injection of the rheumatic patches.

Note no pain-killing, anti-inflammatory, sleep-inducing or tranquillising drugs are used, and there is no injection of the joints themselves.

If patients are closely questioned, you will soon discover, as indeed they themselves have agreed, that the pain they suffer is not persistent and often not particularly severe. What they do then realise is that the fear of not being able to cope with their daily responsibilities is the dominant reason why they seek help. It is almost with joy that more than 80% of patients give up taking any of these drugs, which they took in the first place because they thought they were going to cure them.

Wax baths for the hands and heat elsewhere can do no harm, but equally they do very little good and can be classified in the main as placebo. In contrast, one injection of a relevant rheumatic patch will immediately restore some movement and function with a reduction of pain, even after years of suffering.

All these facts cannot be lightly dismissed because, besides bringing so much relief to the patients, they challenge the use of so many drugs as being superfluous and often so damaging to the patients' health and sometimes causing death [124].

Because of escalating health service costs, it is appropriate to consider the expenditure on all these drugs, the personnel, the equipment, and the space utilised in the physiotherapy departments. The use of the treatment advocated here would render them largely superfluous with a saving to the UK health services I estimate to be at least one billion pounds per annum. (There are over six million people classified as arthritic in the UK.) This could be spent on other departments which are in urgent need of funds. Only a fraction of the amount saved need be devoted to research on the detection of the causative organism, which may prove not very difficult once attention is focused on the primary target of the rheumatic patch.

CHAPTER 6

Allergy and Immunology

INTRODUCTION: ANTIHISTAMINES (D.L.J.F.)

Although not normally thought of in the context of rheumatism therapy, pathologists have discerned for years evidence of degranulated mast cells in the vicinity of rheumatoid joints [30]. Mast cells contain packages of histamine, heparin and other inflammatory mediators, and their function is to liberate these granules under appropriate conditions and so set up a state of acute inflammation. The tissues become distended with fluid, which then flows away down the lymphatics, allowing the lymph nodes to filter and clean up the fluid en route [46]. The process is aggravated by scratching, which is the biological purpose of the itch that accompanies mast cell degranulation.

As we have seen above, the inflammatory response seen in rheumatoid arthritis is puzzling because we cannot perceive an external insult against which the response would be logical. Many doctors therefore have concluded that Nature is making a mistake: the inflammation is inappropriate and paradoxical and should be suppressed. Antihistamines, which partially inhibit the effects of mast cell degranulation, would be a logical weapon to use in the therapeutic armament.

The watching biologist, however, cannot help but feel disquiet about the blunderbuss suppression of a body mechanism that is clearly designed to be doing a job and removing a source of damage from the tissues. Just because we cannot find the insult, it does not prove that there is not one. Nevertheless, we live in the real world. While the suppression of inflammation may well be storing up worse trouble for the patient later on, as the damaging substance builds up to greater and greater levels, we cannot stand idly by awaiting the identification of the putative cause. That might take years, or might never happen, and in the meantime there are people suffering. If we cannot cure the illness, humanity dictates that we should at least attempt to ameliorate the misery while waiting for the breakthrough.

ALLERGY

Many doctors think that allergy is a condition responsible only for sneezes and wheezes, of relatively minor importance as a body mechanism and as a cause of human illness. This is quite wrong. Allergy in fact is a protean system of mechanisms, whose complexities are only just beginning to be worked out. There are at least four different types of allergy, only a small proportion of which involve histamine and most of which are oblivious to antihistamines.

The commonest type—type I hypersensitivity—is the most familiar to patients and doctors. It is mediated by antibodies of the IgE class, which adhere to mast cells and basophils and bring about the familiar picture of mast cell degranulation noted above. Familiar examples of type I diseases would include hay fever and atopic eczema (although this is something of an oversimplification; the interested reader should refer to [47]).

Type II allergy is quite different, being brought about by antibodies of the IgG and IgM classes and involving either the activation of complement or killer cells. The end result is the death of cells, as is seen in some types of haemolytic anaemia.

Type III allergy is brought about by antibodies of the IgG and IgM classes and activated complement. The end results are nephritis, arthritis, fever, and the other manifestations seen most classically in serum sickness.

Type IV allergy is not mediated by antibodies at all but by lymphocytes (T cells) and their products. The end result of type IV allergy is inflammation of the chronic type, in which tissue damage is far more severe than in type I–III allergies and often leaves scarring in its wake. The classic type IV response used to be seen in chronic tuberculosis.

It is a mistake of many doctors to think that 'allergy equals antihistamines' or to behave as though eczema were caused by Betnovate deficiency.

Poisoning

Complicating these immunological pictures further is the role of poisoning. Most of the environmental substances against which an allergic reaction occurs are themselves intrinsically hostile to the host tissues, and (if left to themselves inside the body) would cause damage. Insect stings offer the classic example: pollens and foods are less obvious (but see below). From the biological point of view there is no justification for thinking of 'allergy' and 'immunity' as being in any way separate from each other. They are not. They are two sides of the same coin. Thus, in any illness resulting from the impact of an external insult, the picture is always a composite of two quite different types of process: the direct toxic (poisonous) effect of the insult itself, combined with the inflammatory reaction that the body puts up in self-defence.

Tuberculosis offers again the classic examples. **Miliary** tuberculosis is almost entirely brought about by the direct toxicity of the invading *Mycobacterium tuberculosis*. **Chronic** tuberculosis is almost entirely caused by the body's not-quite-successful attempt to rid itself of the germ. The commonest form of all is **silent infection**; there are a few Mycobacteria somewhere in the body, in hiding, as it were, behind the fibrinous wall of a calcified lymph node, but they have been thoroughly defeated by the immune system and the patient is unaware of having ever been infected since he has never experienced symptoms.

The allergist learns to look for 'insults' in unexpected places. Pollen grains, for example, apparently harmlessly floating about the air in search of a flower to fertilise and occasionally being inhaled and causing hay fever, are actually quite startlingly poisonous [48]. So are many of the plants that humanity habitually uses for food [49]. It is only because Nature has endowed us with a powerful digestive system and many detoxification systems in the liver and lungs that we are (for the most part) unaware of the poisons that we swallow and inhale daily. In our headlong rush for material development we have of course added immeasurably to the toxicity of the environment by polluting soil, air, water and food chains with toxic effluents and chemical pollution, and this perhaps is one reason why allergic illnesses seem to be becoming more and more common [50].

IMMUNOLOGY

Immunology is the study of immunity, that state in which an individual does not become sick, even when exposed to microorganisms that ought to make him sick. Immunity is brought about by a concerted defence effort in the body tissues, and involves cells called **lymphocytes**, a complex set of blood proteins having the collective name **complement**, and **antibodies**. We can tell when an active immune process is under way because the blood white cell count rises, complement is consumed, antibody levels rise, and often the patient suffers from fever, malaise, and the aches and pains associated with inflammation.

All of these things are seen in rheumatoid disease, and it has been accepted for many years that an active immune response of some kind is responsible, but immunity against what? A germ? A chemical? Radiation?

There is an almost embarrassing wealth of circumstantial evidence suggesting that some kind of infection is responsible. Many infections can bring about 'reactive arthritis' as a late sequel. Most notable are the Streptococci, spirochaetes and the organisms of Reiter's disease, but practically every known microorganism has occasionally caused this complication [28, 37, 38]. Then again, dozens of bacteria, ranging from Staphylococci to Salmonellae and the tubercle bacillus (*M. tuberculosis*), have been known to invade joint spaces directly, from the blood or from infections in adjacent tissues, setting up a septic arthritis in the joint. However, in classic rheumatoid disease, in spite of all the signs and symptoms of an active immune process in full spate, it is very rare that specific microorganisms are found in the joint space. To be sure, exacerbations are frequently triggered by an upper respiratory infection, as already noted (see chapter 4), but by the time the joints become inflamed the episode of infection usually appears to have waned. Rheumatoid arthritis, then, fits more easily into our conception of reactive arthritis than that of septic arthritis.

The levels of specific anti-microbial antibodies generally remain unchanged in rheumatoid disease, although the total antibody (immunoglobulin) level is high. Part of this is due to a curious auto-antibody called **rheumatoid factor**. This is an antibody formed against immunoglobulin itself, that is, an antibody directed against the body's own antibodies. Although rather an unsettling concept, anti-antibody antibodies are by no means uncommon. They are found to some extent in all conditions of chronic antibody formation, as for instance an immune response directed against a microorganism that stubbornly refuses to be killed off, and remains within the body for longer than a few weeks. The presence of rheumatoid factor, then, tells us only what we already knew: that there is an active immune response going on, and carrying on for long periods of time. The causative organism or substance (antigen) might either be a very resistant and stubborn microorganism (such as *M. tuberculosis*, or Herpesvirus), or else a component of the body itself.

Experimental animal studies lend some support to both of these notions.

Adjuvant Arthritis

Adjuvant arthritis is a condition seen in rats when they are given subcutaneous injections of certain microorganisms, or of non-living extracts of these organisms. The substance responsible is a bacterial proteoglycan found in several types of bacteria, most notably *M. tuberculosis*. In adjuvant arthritis, as in human rheumatoid disease, there are inflammatory granulomata in various body organs, including the skin. Adjuvant arthritis is tantalisingly similar to human rheumatoid disease, but also has a number of differences. On the whole it is rather more akin to Reiter's arthritis [27].

Collagen Arthritis

Collagen arthritis is an auto-immune condition found in rats and mice that have been immunised with type II collagen (there are five types of collagen in all; type II is the variety found mainly in cartilage). Once again, however, the similarities with human rheumatoid disease are counterbalanced by differences [40], so that on the whole neither of these two experimental animal diseases satisfactorily explains the human condition.

Lectin Arthritis

A third type of experimental arthritis rather more similar to the human rheumatoid joint is that caused by injections of lectins (see below) into the joints of rabbits [55].

We noted above that a foreign substance (antigen) that remained in the body tissues for prolonged periods of time might be either an unusually stubborn microorganism or else a component of the body itself. There is a third possibility. It might be an antigen that *is* removed by the immune system, but is then continually brought back into the body on a daily basis.

DIET

Case reports linking rheumatoid disease with particular food items have appeared sporadically for many years. Parke and Hughes [56] reported a patient whose disease could reliably be made better and worse by the simple expedient of withdrawing milk and dairy products from the diet, then reintroducing them. Pinals [57] noted arthritis in a girl with coeliac disease (gluten-sensitive enteropathy, a disease of the intestines caused by wheat proteins). When gluten was withdrawn, both the intestinal complaint and the arthritis got better. Mäki *et al.* [58] consider the relationship of coeliac disease and arthritis so common that 'arthritis and arthralgia should be included in the list of monosymptomatic forms of coeliac disease'. Such cases are rare (though not perhaps as rare as most doctors think). It is also rare, in allergy practice, to find a patient whose symptoms are caused by one food or substance only; multiple sensitivities are more usual. Nevertheless, the implications of these case reports are intriguing and have prompted some rheumatologists to look more searchingly for evidence of food sensitivity in their patients. One cannot, of course, assume that the culprit foods will be the same in each patient: in allergy circles the old saying that 'one man's meat is another man's poison' is a fundamental daily practicality.

Hicklin *et al.* [59] reported a group of 22 rheumatoid patients, 15 of whom were seropositive (i.e. their blood contained rheumatoid factor). Each patient was put onto a very simple limited diet that avoided grains, milk, potatoes and other foods thought likely to be involved. On this regimen most of the patients felt better—some only slightly but some quite dramatically. A period of 10–18 days elapsed before any improvement became apparent (which offers some argument against a placebo effect). Once improved, the patients were persuaded to reintroduce foods, one at a time, to see whether their arthritis became worse again—again allowing up to two weeks for any deterioration to become apparent. In this way a number of specific foods were implicated, in order of frequency as given in table 2.

Table 2 Specific foods causing relapses of
rheumatoid arthritis [59]

Food	Number of arthritis exacerbations
Grains	14
Pip/nut (fruits)	8
Cheese	7
Egg	5
Milk	4
Beef	4
Chicken	1
Fish	1
Potato	1
Onion	1

This report was, in general, ignored by the medical world because the evidence of non-blind trials (in which the patient knows what treatment he is being given) is weak—the patient's expectations and psychology exert too strong an influence. Six years later, however, Darlington *et al.* [60] reported a rather more scientific trial with statistically acceptable experimental controls (although still without 'blinding' the patient—it is of course very difficult to make sure a patient does not know what he is eating and drinking), and more precise measurements of disease activity. Once again, many patients were found to respond to dietary eliminations and to relapse on reintroduction; once again the incriminated foods were very variable from one patient to another. Stanworth [61] reported that food-sensitive rheumatoids share an abnormal biochemical pattern of α_1-antitrypsin–IgA complex levels. *Starvation* reliably improves rheumatoid symptoms [76].

In general, the foods most often associated with arthritis reactions are more-or-less the same as those that crop up most frequently in association with other food-intolerance syndromes (such as urticaria). The list given above would be a fair representation of what most allergists would expect.

Foods, being (by definition) composed of 'foreign' proteins and carbohydrates, i.e. not derived from the body itself, are antigenic, and evoke an active immune response in the eater. We all have abundant anti-food antibodies in our intestinal juice—they participate, in fact, in the process of digestion [62]. Most of us also have anti-food antibodies in our bloodstreams, evidence that the digestion process is not always 100% efficient. Small fragments of part-digested food molecules usually gain access to the circulation after meals [63]. Foods such as bread and milk are usually taken daily in Western societies, thus fulfilling perfectly the criterion for rheumatoid factor production (see p. 61): that the antigen(s) either refuse to leave the body or else are brought back in every day.

Over the years a number of people have fallen into the trap of thinking that because avoiding certain foods and drinks helped *their* arthritis, the same diet would also benefit others. In recent years the so-called 'Dong diet' has enjoyed a vogue for precisely this reason, only to fail the test of scientific scrutiny [64]. Every patient is different. However, having said that, certain themes do tend to recur. All allergists agree, for instance, that the cultivated grasses—wheat, rye, barley, maize, rice, oats—come at or near the top of the list of foods likely to aggravate arthritis in sensitive individuals. Milk, fruits (especially citrus), nuts, pulses, chocolate, cheese and preservatives are likewise always high on the list. Meats and greens are in general less often troublesome, but there is no such thing as a universally safe food.

LECTINS AND AUTOIMMUNITY

What are Lectins?

Some plants are edible, others poisonous. Some of the most potent homicidal poisons are plant extracts. Many will remember Gyorgi

Markov, the emigré Bulgarian dissident who was assassinated on a London street in 1978 by a man who jabbed his leg with a poison-tipped umbrella. That poison was ricin, a toxic lectin obtained from the seeds of the castor-oil plant, *Ricinus communis*. Ricin is just one example—a particularly deadly example—of a huge range of lectins [65]. All plants have them, but some have more than others, and some lectins are more poisonous than others. Even food vegetables have lectins in them, but usually these are only mildly poisonous. Toxicity within the plant kingdom is a matter of degree.

Lectins are medium-sized protein molecules, sometimes having carbohydrate chains fixed to the sides. They act by binding to the carbohydrate molecules found on the surfaces of cells (the glycoproteins and glycolipids) and the surfaces of other molecules. Once bound, they are reluctant to let go again, behaving in the test-tube rather as antibodies do. There are lectins in wheat and all grains, in legumes, and in all seeds. To a lesser degree they are found in all parts of the plant, including stems, leaves and (when present) tubers. All the plant foods noted above in connection with allergies and arthritis contain lectins. Cheese acquires lectins from the moulds that grow within it. Milk contains lectins, at least at some seasons of the year, derived from the cow's food.

The carbohydrates that lectins bind to are quite specific. There are dozens of different simple carbohydrates (monosaccharides, oligosaccharides, or simply 'sugars'). Glucose is a well-known example (household sugar, sucrose, is a disaccharide made of two linked monosaccharides). Other monosaccharides found in human tissues and cells include galactose, N-acetyl-galactosamine, N-acetyl-glucosamine, fucose and sialic acid. In spite of their fearsome names, these molecules are all very simple structures and resemble each other strongly, so much so that ordinary chemical tests cannot easily distinguish between them. Only lectins (and sometimes antibodies) can tell them apart.

Different lectins have affinities for different monosaccharides. The soybean lectin, for example, is specific for galactose and virtually ignores glucose, even though the structures of the two molecules are so similar. Wheatgerm lectin is specific for N-acetyl-glucosamine (GlcNAc) and oligosaccharides composed of several GlcNAcs linked together.

To recapitulate: of all foods associated with exacerbations of rheumatoid disease, the commonest are grains. Of these, the commonest is wheat. Wheat lectin is specific for GlcNAc. And rheumatoid factor is an auto-antibody against other antibodies.

Antibodies, like lectins, are made up of long protein chains that have carbohydrate side-chains (oligosaccharides) attached. The sugars making up these side-chains, and their sequence in those chains, are known. The antibodies that form the target for rheumatoid factor fall into a class of proteins called immunoglobulin G (IgG). The carbohydrate side-chains of IgG antibodies normally have a galactose molecule at the tip of the chain (the terminal, or immunodominant sugar). The sugar immediately under the terminal galactose (the subterminal sugar) is normally GlcNAc (*N*-acetyl-glucosamine). Now here is the clincher: rheumatoid patients have an inborn weakness in the cells that produce IgG antibodies—they lack the enzyme galactosyltransferase [66]. This means that the carbohydrate side-chains of the IgG antibodies do not terminate with galactose, as they should do, but with the sugar that normally lies underneath, GlcNAc. This is the sugar for which wheatgerm lectin is specific.

Wheatgerm lectin is a very strong molecule. It is not damaged by normal cooking or by digestion [67]. Fresh bread contains appreciable amounts of wheat lectin (D. Freed, unpublished), some of which enters the body circulation each time wheat is eaten. (Stale bread and rusk—which is baked at a much hotter temperature than bread—have much less lectin.) The combination of rheumatoid IgG antibodies, displaying GlcNAc on their side-chains instead of galactose, together with wheatgerm lectin which has a strong affinity for GlcNAc, is irresistible. The lectin must bind to the antibodies (figure 7).

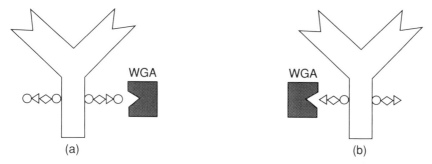

Figure 7 (a) Normal 'complete' IgG antibody. WGA cannot bind to the side-chain sugars because it has no affinity for galactose (○). (b) However, it does have an affinity for GlcNAc (△) and binds strongly.

Rheumatoid people, whenever they eat a food containing wheat, must have some of their IgG antibodies bound by wheat lectin afterwards. The same is true of the cells (plasma cells) that produce these antibodies. Both the cells and their antibodies will have a certain amount of plant protein—wheatgerm lectin—adhering to their surfaces. As such, their surfaces are altered and are likely to attract autoimmune attack.

Autoimmunity

The phenomenon of autoimmunity has fascinated and exasperated scientists for decades. It ought to be impossible—the very word is a contradiction (how can one be immune to oneself?)—yet it exists. Autoimmunity causes juvenile diabetes and thyroid disease, pernicious anaemia and systemic lupus erythematosus. It is associated, as we have seen, with rheumatoid disease. How can it be possible?

Under normal circumstances, body cells are not attacked by autoimmunity because they lack the surface structures known as class II MHC molecules. Only cells displaying both class II molecules *and* antigen can sensitise the immune system (the antigen is held firmly within a cleft in the MHC molecule, so as to be 'presented' to passing lymphocytes) [68]. Plant proteins such as wheatgerm lectin are certainly antigens, but they will not necessarily evoke an immune response unless they are properly presented to the lymphocytes by a cell having a suitable MHC molecule on its surface also.

Most body cells lack class II MHC molecules. However, they can be stimulated to produce them, inappropriately, if exposed to certain substances, notably one called γ-interferon [69]. This substance is produced by lymphocytes in response to virus infections, or in response to certain lectins, including wheatgerm lectin. Having first caused the cell to express aberrant class II molecules [69], the lectin will then bind to them (since class II molecules, like antibodies, have oligosaccharide side-chains attached to their protein cores).

The Lectin Hypothesis of Autoimmunity

A cell that displays an aberrant class II molecule on its surface, and is bound to a plant protein (the lectin that induced the molecule), would form an irresistible focus for autoimmune attack.

We have considered wheatgerm lectin so far in the main, but it should be remembered that all vegetable foods and fruits contain lectins, many of which resist cooking and digestion and gain access to the circulation. The only puzzling feature of the lectin hypothesis, in view of the fact that we all eat lectins most days, is that all of us should by rights have autoimmune diseases.

However, the body has a number of ways in which it can protect itself against lectins, the principal of these being the enormous capacity of the circulating plasma glycoproteins (protein-bound carbohydrates) to 'soak up' lectins. The plasma glycoproteins have a limited lifespan; they are constantly being destroyed by the liver and replaced by new glycoproteins, so there is a constantly replenished pool of glycoproteins available to deal with incoming lectins. In times of extra stress the body produces much more of the glycoproteins, which are then termed 'acute-phase proteins' [70].

If we were to imagine, however, that the 'soaking-up' capacity of the plasma glycoproteins had been exceeded, so that once again there were free lectins in the circulation, the next barrier would be posed by the connective tissue matrix. The connective tissue matrix (see pp. 91, 93–94) is made up largely of glycosaminoglycans (GAGs), which are composed of long chains of sugars—perfect targets for lectins. Only after the capacity of the body GAG matrix had been overwhelmed would the spillover lectins be available to attack cells.

Other Properties of Lectins

Many lectins are polyclonal mitogens; that is, they can induce lymphocytes to enter a phase of multiplication by repeated binary fission, so that instead of one cell there will be, after a few hours, two cells, then four, then eight, then 16, then 32, and so on until the process overruns the body or is halted by one of the body's regulatory mechanisms. Not only lymphocytes but also gut epithelial cells [71] and epidermal cells [72] are susceptible to the mitogenic action of lectins. Another intriguing property of certain lectins is **mast cell degranulation**; that is, they stimulate the liberation within the body tissues of large quantities of histamine and other inflammatory mediators [73].

Both mitogenesis and mast cell degranulation are features of the body's immune defence against invading microorganisms. What lectins do is to 'fool' the immune system into thinking that the body is under microbial attack, so that it responds vigorously in defence against the imagined invasion.

Rheumatoid patients have an inherent weakness in both respects. Rheumatoid lymphocytes are less able than ordinary lymphocytes to respond appropriately to antigenic and mitogenic stimuli [74, 75]. Rheumatoid patients also have an unfortunate predilection to generate auto-antibodies of the IgE class [77]. (IgE antibodies are those responsible normally for triggering mast cell degranulation; they are the hallmark of 'allergic' reactions such as hay fever and eczema. One of the intriguing minor side-effects of lectins is their ability to divert an ongoing immune response into IgE production [78, 79].)

There is a fascinating two-way interaction between lectins and microorganisms. In one direction, many germs are themselves lectins— famous examples include the influenza virus and *Bordetella pertussis*, the germ that causes whooping cough—and these germs themselves are known to stimulate IgE production. In the other direction, certain germs that prefer to set up a cosy commensal relationship with their host's cells, lying dormant for the host's lifespan (these include most of the herpes viruses, measles virus, and the bacteria of tuberculosis and brucellosis, not to mention the AIDS virus) can be 'brought out of hiding' when the host cells are exposed to lectins [80–82], so that there is an acute disease reaction instead of the low level insidious illness that the germs would prefer to cause.

Lectins and Connective Tissues

In the main we shall consider the behaviour of wheatgerm lectin (WGA; the 'A' denotes 'agglutinin') in this section, because (a) there are simply too many lectin–tissue interactions reported in the literature for them to be sensibly reviewed here, (b) wheat lectin is particularly likely to reach the body tissues after eating because it is unusually resistant to cooking and digestion, (c) its interactions with human tissues have been better investigated than those of any other lectin because it is cheap and easy to obtain, and (d) wheat is the one food most strongly associated clinically with acute exacerbations of arthritis. Nevertheless, you should bear in mind that WGA is but one out of thousands of lectins, and many others could equally well be involved in disease causation (these would include lectins of viral origin also, such as influenza virus lectin).

In the test-tube, WGA binds to most of the components of connective tissue and principally to certain glycosaminoglycans (GAGs): keratan sulphate [83–85], chondroitin sulphate [86], heparan sulphate [87] and the link proteins of proteoglycans [88]. It also binds, although less strongly, to elastin and collagen [89]. Both cartilage and bone are susceptible [90–93] as well as muscle, skin and subcutaneous connective tissues [94, 95] (because of their high heparan sulphate content). Many of the *cells* of connective tissue are also affected by WGA, including chondrocytes [96], synovial lining cells [97, 99], and, most importantly, fibroblasts [98].

The fibroblast is the central enigma of **rheumatoid nodules**. Why, in the centre of a nodule, in the presence of a patch of tissue degeneration which ought to be an irresistible focus for inflammation, do the fibroblasts not invade the patch and begin their task of repair? Why do they instead line up at the borders of the nodule as if they wanted to get in but were being forbidden to enter? Why do rheumatoid nodules swell up with GAG-rich gel? Why does osteoporosis (thinning of the bone) appear at the edge of the rheumatoid joint right at the start of the inflammation within the joint? There is now a wealth of evidence pointing to lectins, and particularly WGA, as the most plausible key to these enigmatic features.

WGA at certain dose levels (and several other lectins) stimulates the synthesis and release of GAGs and collagenase (an enzyme that breaks down collagen) from fibroblasts at the same time as slowing down their protein and DNA metabolism and their speed of migration [100–108].

The effects of WGA on bone have not so far been studied, but three legume lectins (kidney bean, jackbean and soya) have been reported [92, 93]. Of particular interest is the kidney bean lectin; it stimulates osteoclasts (the cells responsible for nibbling away and removing unwanted bone), so that the bone becomes thinner (i.e. osteoporosis) and (in the growing animal) grows more slowly. Soybean lectin has no effect on bone cells, but jackbean lectin had the opposite effect of inhibiting osteoclasts (this, however, is of less compelling interest since the jackbean is not a human food). At the whole-animal level arthritis was induced in rabbits by a single injection of lectin into the joint. The most powerful lectin in this experiment was lentil; WGA was rather less effective [55, 109].

THE LECTIN HYPOTHESIS

We are now able to use this varied information to construct a general picture of one likely cause of rheumatoid disease. The hypothesis fits with all known clinical, scientific and dietary data, as well as with the observations as set out in chapters 3 and 5. If the hypothesis is true, it could be exploited therapeutically.

Lectin — mainly but not exclusively from wheat and other grains — enters the intestine whenever we eat the relevant foods. The amount of lectin entering depends on how thoroughly the food was baked beforehand, and the other processing stages it has been through. Much of the lectin is eliminated or destroyed in the gut and liver but some — perhaps only a small percentage — evades destruction and enters the bloodstream.

This, in most people most of the time, will be as far as the lectin gets because of the blood glycoproteins, which have a huge capacity for soaking up lectins. Some people, however, have a more limited capacity, perhaps (as in the case of the rheumatoid patients' IgG antibodies, noted on p. 65) because the glycoproteins are imperfectly formed by a genetically deficient enzyme.

Alternatively, a person with normal blood glycoproteins might be overwhelmed by a really big intake of wheat lectin (probably this happens from time to time in most people). In these cases, excess lectin spills over from the blood into surrounding tissues and is taken up by the GAGs of the connective tissue matrix (and to some extent by the collagen and elastin). The connective tissue of the skin, having a high content of heparan sulphate, would be particularly attractive to WGA. Cartilage would also be attractive, in this case because of its keratan sulphate.

Connective tissue that has absorbed lectin is likely to become stiffer [110], causing a realignment of stress trajectories (see p. 94 for the physical properties of composite materials) and the paradoxical weakening of the tissue that realignment leads to. Under conditions of everyday movement, minor damage is likely to occur at these areas, with micro-splitting of the connective tissues and tenderness. Sudden big stresses (such as falls or sports injuries) might cause tissue failure on a larger scale, with more severe pain and perhaps bruising.

A body tissue with plant protein firmly attached must attract the attention of the immune system ('autoimmunity'), and phagocytes and fibroblasts will be attracted to the site. This will especially be so if there is some tissue damage, as then the powerfully chemoattractant kinins and complement components will be brought into play. However, as the inflammatory cells approach the centre of the area the concentration of WGA rises, eventually reaching a level at which the fibroblasts can no longer crawl [105]. They will have no choice but to stop moving, attracted by the chemotactic influence at the centre of the patch but immobilised by lectin, eventually forming a circle or palisade around the periphery. The same WGA concentration, however, would at the same time stimulate collagenase and GAG secretion by the fibroblasts, pumping up the tissue with fluid and cutting the 'ropes' of collagen that normally keep connective tissues internally anchored. A **rheumatoid nodule** is thus formed. However, what of rheumatic patches?

Here is the missing link in our hypothetical chain of events. How do we explain the increased and haphazard deposition of collagen seen in rheumatic patches? Does WGA also stimulate collagen deposition by fibroblasts, perhaps at a different dose level from the one needed to stimulate GAG secretion, or later on? At the time of writing we do not know, although Dr. U. Schumacher at the University of Munich is actively engaged in research that will eventually provide the result. We do not therefore yet know whether the lectin hypothesis encompasses the formation of true rheumatic patches as well as rheumatoid nodules. The limit of our predictive power is that WGA-encrusted connective tissues are likely to be stiffer than normal tissues.

What of the joints? Here we become more speculative. One could envisage that the joints might be subjected to extra stresses by rheumatic patches in connective tissue or muscle, just as the tension at the apex of a tent would be increased if we tied extra knots in the guy ropes. Eventually the fabric at the tent apex would be liable to tear, even though the cause of the extra tension were far away. (Injecting salicylate—or, using the tent analogy, cutting some of the knotted guy ropes—would release some of the tension.) One could expect joint pain to occur, even without actual damage to the joint surfaces, and this would be reinforced by the reflex muscle spasm that automatically sets in to protect painful soft-tissue lesions [32]. Misaligned stress trajectories in connective tissues, reinforced by muscle spasm, eventually distort the alignment of the spinal vertebrae [32], so setting the whole structure rigidly into a slightly more comfortable, but eventually more damaging, posture.

Once lectin starts to spill over into the joint cavities themselves, inflammation would be initiated by mast cell activation [73] and perhaps complement activation [111], platelet aggregation [112, 113] and coagulation of synovial fluid with fibrin deposition. These, of course, are precisely what the pathologist perceives as the earliest signs of rheumatoid arthritis, and precisely what Stillmark noticed, 100 years ago, in his first observations on lectins [114]. Since the GAG level in synovial fluid is low in comparison with connective tissue, the lectin level is unlikely to build up to levels that would inhibit the influx of inflammatory cells. Lectins adsorbed to subjacent bone would stimulate osteoclasts [93] and cause the paradoxical osteoporosis noted above. Elastin with lectin attached (although this has not been experimentally verified) would probably lose its elastic properties and we may therefore expect to see relaxation of ligaments and joint capsule (and we do).

Thus far I have mainly concerned myself with wheat lectin, but it should be remembered that most foods of plant origin contain lectins (especially the starchy foods such as grains, legumes and root crops), to say nothing of the invasive lectins such as those attached to viruses and bacteria. The effects of the various lectins could in some cases be additive, and in other cases mutually cancelling, leading to a great variety of possible outcomes. Another caveat is that I have described the four lectin-absorbing compartments of the body—plasma, connective tissues, joints and lymphocytes—as if they were strictly consecutive, so that one must be filled up completely before any spillover occurs into the next, like waterfalls in a cascade. In real life one would expect considerable blurring of the margins, since affinity phenomena never reach complete saturation.

OSTEOARTHRITIS

The pathology of the osteoarthritic joint is quite different from that of the rheumatoid joint, and has led most workers to conclude that there are two quite distinct disease processes. In osteoarthritis the first changes seen in the joint are focal patches of depletion of cartilage proteoglycans (even though proteoglycan production by local chondrocytes may actually be increased), followed by a characteristic type of roughening of the cartilage surface known as **fibrillation**. Fissures and ulceration of the cartilage follow, with compensatory proliferation of chondrocyte clusters. The collagen fibrils become thickened and irregular. Capillaries from subjacent bone invade the tidemark region leading to new bone formation (osteophytes), which parallels the denudation of cartilage. Hence the frequent remark that osteoarthritis is a consequence of 'wear and tear', whereas rheumatoid arthritis is the result of chronic inflammation. However, if this were so we would expect osteoarthritis to be a relentlessly progressive condition, unresponsive to anti-inflammatory drugs, and this is not entirely so.

Bill Fox is adamant that osteoarthritis and rheumatoid arthritis alike respond to his treatments, and I have argued above that rheumatoid disease bears all the hallmarks of dietary lectin causation. Could the lectin hypothesis be expanded to accommodate osteoarthritis also?

I have already mentioned that the lectin WGA (wheatgerm lectin) exerts a dual effect on human fibroblasts, stimulating their GAG secretion but inhibiting their motility and general metabolism. I used this datum in building up a lectin hypothesis for the formation of rheumatoid nodules. In fact the paper that I cited deserves far closer attention than might seem apparent [100], and the reader is recommended to read it.

It will be seen (figure 8) that WGA has two opposite effects on GAG secretion: at moderate concentration it is enhanced, as noted above, but

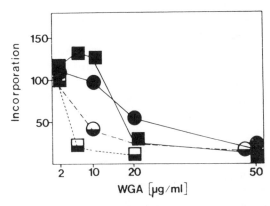

Figure 8 Synthesis and secretion of glycosaminoglycans (■), proteins (●) and DNA (□) by isolated human fibroblasts incubated in the test tube with wheat lectin (WGA) at various concentrations [100]. Reproduced with the permission of the editors.

at higher concentrations it is inhibited together with the other indices of metabolic activity. If fibroblasts are exposed over a period of time to a gradually increasing WGA concentration, the GAG secretion rises at first but after a time is strongly inhibited. Precisely the same pattern is seen in human and experimental osteoarthritis [115], and lectin-stimulated cells, both monocytes and chondrocytes, dissolve cartilage [116, 117] or disorganise its development [118]. I think the answer to my question is clear: yes, food lectins could well be involved, on the basis of what we already know about their behaviour *in vitro*, in the aetiology of both rheumatoid disease and osteoarthritis. The difference is merely one of dose level, osteoarthritis requiring a rather higher dose of WGA. Several lectins have an affinity for human cartilage and chondrocytes [119], with higher binding to fibrillated cartilage (i.e. in the early stages of osteo-arthritis).

Bill Fox has already expressed his positive views on allergy based on pure clinical evidence. This chapter has tried to provide the current scientific thinking in this field and we share a great measure of agreement.

CHAPTER 7

Other Forms of Rheumatism and Differential Diagnosis

INTRODUCTION   (W.W.F.)

Up to this point, the main emphasis in diagnosis and treatment has been on rheumatoid arthritis. Its relationship with pre-arthritic states and osteoarthritis has been defined, with the rheumatic patch as the common factor. Let us now consider a number of commonly accepted clinical descriptions of disease which stand in isolation, implying that they are not related to other known forms of rheumatic disease: headaches, migraine, frozen shoulder, sprains and strains, tennis or golfers' elbow, and low back pain.

HEADACHES

These vary in both their frequency and their severity. The common location is at the base of the skull, temporal and frontal areas. In women they tend to be worse during the premenstrual stage and improve postmenstrually. It is extremely rare to find a case which does not have other symptoms of rheumatic involvement elsewhere in the body. Because most sufferers take aspirin or similar drugs for their relief, the natural history of the headache is lost.

Physical examination of the head and neck frequently shows limitation of movement, sometimes with pain, in one or more directions. Some pain is induced or made worse when attempts are made to increase the range of movement of the head and neck. By using the methods described previously, rheumatic patches will be located at the back of the neck from the base of the skull down to the fourth thoracic vertebra level. Injection of these patches with sodium salicylate will either abolish the headache or reduce it quite considerably within two minutes.

Patients frequently realise, to their great surprise, that their heads feel much lighter and clearer. Only then do they realise that, even when they had no headache, there was a dullness which was accepted as normal because they had forgotten (or never knew) what a normal head was like. A further bonus was later noted by many: now a strain was absent when using their eyes—again they had forgotten what normality was.

For this reason all rheumatic patients are warned not to have their eyes tested when the disease is active and particularly when a headache is present. This precaution reduces the number of disappointed people who find the spectacles do not help the headaches or eyestrain for very long. The prognosis in all these cases of headache is precisely the same as the arthritic ones. They thus become an understandable diagnosis as part of the chronic rheumatic syndrome.

MIGRAINE

This is a more severe form of headache, with its own well-known characteristics. Allergy appears to be a major factor and this aspect should receive detailed attention. The physical findings on examination are the same as in headaches but the patches are more widespread. The response to treatment is just as good, providing that all the patches, some of which are lateral to the mid-line, are fully treated.

FROZEN SHOULDER

History and examination follow the usual pattern. In this condition, rheumatic patches will be found spreading from levels of the third thoracic vertebra down to at least the sixth and possibly to the eighth. There will also be further large rheumatic patches distally depending on the length and severity of the condition and also the kind of treatment the patient has been given. Obviously, in the earlier stages, the patches will be smaller and less in number, and therefore more amenable to treatment.

If, however, the patient has been treated with physiotherapy, as is almost always the case, the patches will be widespread, as a result of massage and movement, for this serves only to spread inflammation along the connective tissue which, in turn, becomes increasingly adherent to the skin above it.

Examination in these cases will reveal so many widespread rheumatic patches that you will readily appreciate there is a lot of work to be done before real improvement is manifest. By the judicious choice of relevant patches, it is possible to demonstrate some limited improvement at the first or second treatment. In a long-standing case, this is very important, because it will give the patients some hope and encouragement, where before there was none. It is a psychological lift which they badly need.

SPRAINS AND STRAINS

Early rheumatic cases declare themselves quite frequently by recurring sprains or strains affecting the limbs or back.

Let us consider two very common cases which, for ease in presentation, I shall address as to the patients.

You are doing a simple job which you have done hundreds of times before, lifting a pan off the stove or using a screwdriver. Suddenly, your wrist gets painful, and you think 'Ah! I have sprained it.' You have to stop what you are doing, rest the wrist, perhaps bandage it; in a day or two it is better, and you forget about it. If it is very painful and does not settle fairly quickly, you go to the doctor. He confirms it is a sprain, gives you some liniment or whatever, and in due course you get better. The real diagnosis and the question of rheumatism have never arisen.

The same confusion can arise when an ankle is affected. In this case, you think you have tripped over a stair or pavement, when in fact your foot has given way because of a sudden rheumatic attack. The same story as for the wrist is repeated. Of course, you can trip over a stair or a pavement and do yourself an injury when you have no rheumatism. In these cases, you can get up and start walking normally if there is no severe injury, otherwise there is pain, bruising and swelling to confirm the real injury. None of these do you find if rheumatism is the cause. You may, of course, trip because of rheumatism and cause a more severe injury to the ankle area with bruising and swelling. Now you suffer the effect of two conditions — the rheumatic condition and the injury. These are the cases which take much longer than expected to get better because the injury aggravates the rheumatism, and the rheumatism delays the normal recovery process. The recovery is even further delayed when it is not realised that there may be rheumatic patch present in the area, because the next stage in the treatment for this injury is heat, massage and exercises. The heat can do little harm, but the massage and exercises will only aggravate the inflamed rheumatic patch. These kinds of problems, whether affecting the wrist, elbow, ankle or knee, are common.

It should be noted that sprains and strains are so common that they are referred to in a Government report [18]. It showed an increase in absence from work from 9.4 days per 60 men in 1954 to over 50 days in 1980. Similarly, nervous tension (discussed in chapter 5) and headaches increased from 9 to 60 days, while arthritis increased from 43 to 125 days. If the first two categories had been recognised as rheumatic in origin it would have provided a simple logical relationship to all three.

Tennis Elbow

The problem in tennis elbow (which also applies to golfers) arises because the symptoms of pain and restriction of movement appear to occur when actually playing. They are often first seen by the GP or a physiotherapist. X-rays are sometimes taken to exclude bony injury. As these almost always prove negative, the unscientific and unsubstanti- ated assumption is then made that some tendinous or muscle fibres have been torn. Now, equally unscientific treatment is instituted: heat, which can do no harm; rest, which is helpful; or massage and exercises which do nothing but harm. Because the persistent failure of these methods has become all too obvious, many are now treated with an injection of steroids into the supposedly damaged area. This causes immediate acute pain for some, followed by relief, while others, with little or no pain, also experience relief.

For those with severe pain on injection, it can be surmised that the fluid has inadvertently been injected into a rheumatic patch and hence the immediate improvement. The cases where there is no severe pain on injection suggest that the rheumatic patch has been missed equally inadvertently. The improvement shown by both for a variable period of time is due entirely to the general effect of the steroid in suppressing the symptoms.

Now let us consider a similar case where a detailed and careful history is taken, followed by a physical examination. There is, without exception, a history of other rheumatic manifestations such as growing pains, backache, stiff neck. Many of the patients will actually have had such symptoms when they went to play tennis or golf. Some will recall a sore throat, or what they erroneously call a cold, a few days prior to the incident.

Examination will reveal rheumatic patches not only at the site of the pain but also elsewhere in the arm or other parts of the body.

The true diagnosis is now fairly obvious. A sudden exacerbation of a rheumatic patch occurred while playing — this was the cause of the pain and not the physical movement; in fact, the pain inhibited any further movement.

When you think about it, as I have done in the past before the rheumatic patch was identified, why should the repetition of a simple action — say in hitting a tennis ball or swinging a golf club — suddenly give rise to torn muscles or tendinous fibres in a healthy person who has been doing exactly the same movements most of their active life? It would seem even less likely in a professional player. Given these facts, the treatment, including advice, is then logically based on the rheumatic syndrome and injection of relevant patches.

However, at the time of the alleged injury, the disease is likely to be in its active phase. This means that long-lasting improvement cannot be expected from the first injection of the rheumatic patches, but the period of response will be a valuable guide to the activity of the disease process.

Treatment

The most important step in treatment at this stage is rest for the affected limb — no massage or exercises. The general treatment outlined for all rheumatic conditions, which includes aspirin for a few days, should be initiated. It should also be realised that the body is actively engaged in developing its own resistance and repairing structural damage to the tissues. That is why patients recover from their diseases and injuries. The function of the medical profession should be first to establish the correct diagnosis and then to consider in what way they can assist the healing process. The outstanding examples of these basic requirements can be seen in the surgical, nursing and retraining schedules adopted in the treatment of genuine diagnosable injuries sustained in accidents. Their achievements are beyond praise, because clinical diagnosis and scientific progress work in harmony.

Even in this area, some cases do not make the expected improvement. Pain and limitation of movement persist longer than usual. Physiotherapy and exercises are continued with renewed vigour but still the patient complains. Drugs are usually introduced at this point, aspirin or stronger versions including anti-inflammatories, and, if the patient is suspected of being overanxious, tranquillisers are added.

As many accidents involve claims for damages and compensation, these persistent cases become the object of suspicion as possible malingerers. Without the knowledge of the rheumatic patch, what else would the consultant think? Have they not done everything possible for the patient? Regimens which are so successful for the majority cannot be wrong for the minority — it must be the patient who is at fault!

Here is reprinted from *Arthritis and Allied Conditions* a case which illustrates all the points raised [7].

Case Study 1

February 28, 1968: L.C.E.; male age 24

Complains of pain and weakness right index finger. Pain in lumbar area, right ischeal area and right outer aspect of hip, mostly when sitting and walking. Pain in neck with some headaches at frequent intervals.

Stiff back in the morning, improves with movement but recurs during day especially after sitting for over 20–30 minutes.

History
June 1967: involved in a motor accident. Damage to jaws with loss of teeth. Fracture head of second metacarpal right index finger. Linear fracture right pelvis with flake of bone in right hip.

By the time he saw me the metacarpal fracture was healed but the finger was still painful and weak.

The spicule of bone in the hip joint was absorbed and the linear fracture totally disappeared. He still complained of pain as described above.

Treatment after discharge from ward was heat, exercise and massage three times weekly, with various drugs.

He was referred to me because his condition was worsening and he always felt much worse after treatment.

Examination showed
1. Marked tenderness right neck lateral to C.3.4.5.6.
2. Tenderness, weakness and some thickening right index M.C. joint. Tenderness right middle finger M.C. joint.
3. Tender areas along lumbar spine, right ischeal region and outer aspect of right hip. Severe pain on flexion of right hip beyond 45°.

All these symptoms and signs indicated a generalised rheumatic involvement of the soft tissues brought on by the accident. I expressed this opinion and suggested that unless he was adequately treated arthritis would be inevitable.

I then saw him in consultation with a physician and a little later with an orthopaedic surgeon, both representing the insurance company.

They both totally rejected my diagnosis and insisted that he was exaggerating his symptoms which would improve with adequate damages.

The patient, however, did have treatment and within 2 years he was very greatly improved in his general health and the severity of the pains. At this stage the conditions was as follows:

1. The finger continued to be weak but pain had lessened while the middle finger was very much better.
2. Headaches were not as severe but there was continuing discomfort in the neck.
3. He was walking better with a much slighter limp but still had pain in the hip and back which did not allow him to sit comfortably.

September 1971: I saw him in consultation with the same orthopaedic surgeon. He still persisted in his opinion that there was nothing wrong with the neck or lumbar spine, that there was no physical explanation for the weakness in his finger and pain in the hip, and that it was all exaggerated.

As a result, the patient was offered puny compensation and ceased to attend for further treatment, because he was worried about the account which he might not be able to pay. However, he said he was so much improved that he would try to carry on.

September 1974: I saw him in consultation with the same orthopaedic surgeon. The patient had maintained his improvement but still had the same residual symptoms. A further X-ray at this time showed early osteoarthritis in cervical 5 and some deterioration in the hip joint. It took six years to vindicate the patient's honesty, my diagnosis and prognosis. Needless to say, a substantial settlement was agreed on the morning of the court hearing.

Comment
This case is included, not to denigrate the physician or the orthopaedic surgeon, but because it highlights some very important points made in the text.

1. With no previous history of rheumatism it must be assumed that the shock and the accident initiated the disease process.
2. The disease process took six years before the first signs of arthritis in the neck were demonstrable by X-ray. If you use X-ray films as the cornerstone of evidence in developing arthritis, then all the other symptoms of pain, discomfort, loss of movement, etc. are not correctly evaluated. This was obviously true of the surgeon and the physician in this case.
3. A real understanding of the rheumatic process enables you to ask the appropriate questions and to direct your examination to the affected areas and thus to arrive at the correct diagnosis.
4. Unless the right diagnosis is made, the patient is in danger of being misjudged and mistreated. When the doctor does not understand this disease process, the evidence of organic disease is not appreciated, and the inevitable and easy diagnosis of tension or neurosis is made

or, as in this case, malingering. This patient had been given analgesics and tranquillisers prior to seeing me. They became quite unnecessary the moment correct diagnosis and treatment were begun.

As a corollary to this case and also to underline the contention that pain is primarily and mainly caused by the rheumatic patch and hardly ever by the arthritis, consider the following case.

Case Study 2

November 21, 1983: T.R.; male age 62, foreman steel fitter

Complaint
April 24, 1982: accident at work which caused the right ankle to become painful and swollen. X-ray showed advanced osteoarthritis in the right ankle and early osteoarthritis in the left ankle.

History
Right ankle sprain at work seven years ago. X-ray negative. Cleared up with rest in three weeks. Has worked ever since without complaint.

Details of the treatment and opinions on the recent accident are as follows.

Opinion: August 20, 1982; Hospital Clinic Registrar FRCS
T.R. suffered a severe sprain of his ankle in the accident which has necessitated some five weeks in plaster, four weeks using crutches and partial weight bearing and two months of physiotherapy. In spite of this intensive treatment he still has a painful ankle with restricted movements and is unable to walk without a stick. There is no doubt he has injured this right ankle in the past and had degenerative changes in the ankle with ossicles and early arthritis. The recent ankle sprain has doubtless exacerbated his arthritic ankle. I think with intensive physiotherapy and rehabilitation T.R.'s symptoms will be improved greatly although I fear the range of movements in this ankle will always be restricted.

Opinion: July 31, 1983; Consultant Orthopaedic Surgeon
This patient had an osteoarthritic right ankle long before the accident under consideration as shown by the marked X-ray changes. It will be reasonable in view of his age and his overweight to allow him aching and discomfort from the date of the accident (April 21, 1982) until about January 1983. By then any symptoms from the accident would have

settled and if he still had symptoms they would be due to the osteoarthritic change.

Opinion: October 28, 1983; Hospital Clinic Registrar FRCS
As a result of the accident T.R. suffered a severe sprain of the ankle which necessitated some five weeks in plaster followed by a long period of rehabilitation and physiotherapy. In spite of these measures he has been left with restricted movements at the ankle and subtalar joints, the subtalar joints being very painful. There is also tenderness over the lateral ligament of the ankles. He had suffered a previous injury to the ankle and there were marked degenerative changes present in the ankle at the time of the accident. The accident did, however, cause a serious exacerbation of his arthritic symptoms. It is now more than a year since his accident and I think it highly unlikely that any further improvement will take place. The disability he has now must be considered permanent, but due to the progression of the degenerative process rather than the injury sustained in April 1982.

None of these reports mentions the low back syndrome which came to light in a DHSS report of November 3, 1983, when assessing his industrial accident claim. They did not consider it relevant to his disability.

Examination
Examination demonstrated the presence of rheumatic patches in the lower back, which had been subjected to enormous strain during the accident, and confirmed the ankle condition.

Treatment
Injection of the low back rheumatic patches produced immediate improvement. Three treatments in eight days abolished all his symptoms. He remained free of all pain and disability for the next three years, since when I have no reports.

A consideration of his history indicates that the 'severe ankle sprain' seven years ago while at work was his first attack of rheumatism, involving a rheumatic patch in the lower back which affected the right ankle. It settled down after three weeks of rest and no further symptoms were experienced in the ankle. However, he did become aware of intermittent pain and discomfort in the low back area which he chose to ignore. He climbed 100 ft trees and worked long hours with never a murmur about his ankle until this accident.

The details of this accident disclosed that his right foot was trapped under a steel girder lying on the floor, at the moment when a spring loaded girder he was manipulating on the wall, at head height, flew from his grasp and hit his forehead with great force gashing the scalp and forcing his whole body backwards with hyperextension of the lumbar spinal area. This must have caused severe strain on the connective tissues in that area, where we now know there were rheumatic patches.

My report concluded that this accident was the cause of all his symptoms. Without it his arthritic ankles may never have caused any marked symptoms beyond a very gradual lessening of ankle movement which few people notice as they become older. It is, however, possible that his lower back pain may recur intermittently.

The patient's story was as fundamentally sound and true in this accident as it was in the first 'accident' seven years before. The orthopaedic opinions could no longer be sustained and a rapid and highly satisfactory settlement of the injury claim was achieved. (It was equally important that the patient, a life-long dedicated worker, resented the medical implications that he was a malingerer and seeking unjustified recompense.)

LOW BACK PAIN

Low back pain is not a diagnosis, it is a vague description of a symptom, and until this symptom is clinically analysed it does not seem feasible to reach an understanding of, or a solution to, the problem.

Clinical History

It can begin as an acute form of lumbago which gradually subsides but in some cases there is a residual discomfort, which comes and goes over the years but eventually settles as a chronic nagging ache or pain, made worse by certain movements or positioning in a chair or bed. Many develop in the same way but without an acute onset.

It is quite often attributed to a severe strain or sprain to the ligaments or muscles in the lower back, while at work, strenuous exercise or playing games. Many of these cases quickly improve with rest, physiotherapy and exercise. Those which fail to resolve become patients with persistent low back pain. It is extremely rare to find low back pain of long standing occurring without a history of other symptoms such as pain in the dorsal or cervical region, discomfort or aching in the arms and legs. Frequently the onset of low back pain blocks out a previous pain or discomfort in the dorsal or cervical region and vice versa. This is a very striking feature in rheumatoid arthritis. Furthermore, low back pain can suddenly disappear or reappear without apparent reason. It behaves in exactly the same way as any other feature of those diseases such as arthritis of the hip to which it is closely related, both anatomically and symptomatically.

In 40 years of dealing with the chronic rheumatic diseases, I have found low back pain, at any stage, to be a very common episodic symptom in rheumatoid and osteoarthritis. Because rheumatoid arthritis develops relatively quickly and has so many painful and obvious pathologies, the back pain does not often obtrude itself in the minds of the patient or the physician.

In osteoarthritis, which develops quite slowly over three or four decades, back pain can be a common and dominant feature of the disease. However, a detailed clinical study will reveal the other features referred to previously.

By analysing all the movements of the lumbar spine and noting where and when the pain is modified, the rheumatic patches will be revealed very quickly. The response to treatment will follow the same pattern as all the other cases.

The fact that low back pain is primarily studied and treated by orthopaedic surgeons indicates that it is not considered to be an inflammatory disease or related to rheumatic conditions. Research into this problem is directed, therefore, to posture, injury and maladjustments of the lumbar vertebral column.

It is quite understandable that orthopaedic specialists will have difficulty in believing the osteoarthritis of the lumbar spine can have an inflammatory basis. There is absolutely no evidence in the joints to support such a view and it appears to be a straightforward case of wear and tear.

It is even more obvious that, where a history of sprain, strain or injury to the back has been established, the very idea of an inflammatory origin would have no chance of acceptance.

This is why the persistent failure to cope with the problem is exactly the same as the others. Clinical medicine, which ought to provide the guidelines on which research is based, has been supplanted by what can be described only as misguided science.

The cardinal error of the doctors is their assumption that the pain emanates from a primary injury or fault in the bone structure or the joints between them. Engineers and scientists have collaborated with doctors to try to solve the problem, possibly on the basis that the spinal column of bones together with the pelvis constitute a supportive structure which maintains the integrity of the body in much the same way as a steel or concrete bridge span and its columns support the traffic which uses it or, even more easily understood, the steel skeleton of a building on which everything else depends.

Such a concept is probably incorrect and there may be quite a different mechanism as to how the body maintains stability. This is more fully discussed in chapter 8.

DIFFERENTIAL DIAGNOSIS

The late Sir William Osler, that great clinical diagnostician, asserted that doctors in any department of medical practice could never be considered efficient unless they fully understood all the variants in syphilitic disease. He pointed out that this disease could mimic so many other ailments and complaints that it must be ruled out before any other diagnosis was made.

Taking into account that Sir William Osler was a consultant whose practice was restricted to hospitals and consultations, he would be referring to those patients with major diseases in his own practice. He would therefore have little or no experience of the problems described in this book. However, what he said about syphilis can now be applied, with even greater emphasis, to the chronic rheumatic diseases, and specifically to the rheumatic patch. Its dominance in the causation and treatment has already been demonstrated in those conditions wrongly designated as diseases, when they are really only symptoms. There are many other cases which never go to the rheumatic departments because their symptoms suggest diseases located in the abdominal or chest cavities.

As far back as 1965 the failure to explain some of the 'abdominal' problems had received considerable attention. This letter from Mr. Daintree Johnson, a surgeon at the Royal Free Hospital, London, appeared in the *Lancet* in 1965.

ABDOMINAL PAIN OF SPINAL ORIGIN

SIR, — It is a common experience in surgical clinics to encounter patients with very persistent subcostal pain which defies diagnosis in whom physical examination is unproductive and the usual investigations unrewarding. In some the pain is made worse by certain postures, such as that apt to be assumed in an armchair; or by jolting as while descending stairs, when the spring ligament is less able to fill its usual shock-absorber role.

The pain tends to occur in attacks lasting days or weeks and responds only to aspirin. These patients are commonly referred for "dyspepsia" or "? gallstones", presumably because of the position of the pain, but many of them must surely be cases of dorsal prolapsed intervertebral disc.

I am at a loss how to treat them.

London, N.6.   H. DAINTREE JOHNSON.

Unable to make a diagnosis, he suggested the possibility of a prolapsed disc, a condition which was then greatly in fashion with the medical profession. Time and improved radiological techniques made such a diagnosis untenable in many cases. It also coincided with the stage in my researches when the rheumatic patch was emerging as a clinical entity. This offered a rational explanation of all those symptoms which were not understood and not due to prolapsed disc.

In *Arthritis and Allied Conditions* [7] I gave details of cases where the symptoms of a prolapsed disc were mimicked by a rheumatic patch and which were abolished by its injection with sodium salicylate. Similar dramatic results were obtained in a variety of vague abdominal symptoms where the question of a prolapsed disc did not arise.

Perhaps 'mimicked' is not the most appropriate word. Any experienced clinician would have no difficulty in diagnosing the common diseases associated with this area. It is precisely because symptoms remain unexplained that frustration sets in and multiple investigations which can be used only for known diseases are undertaken. Not unexpectedly, they prove that the clinician was right in the first place: 'It defies diagnosis.'

Unexplained low back pain is frequently investigated for a possible carcinoma of the colon, particularly when associated with constipation. The constipation has usually been caused by the drugs the patient has been taking for the pain relief. Where the pain is located in the kidney region, similar and unpleasant expensive investigations are instituted.

These are some of the possible diseases 'mimicked by' the rheumatic patch, whose reality or absence can be so easily established.

There are those cases where the whole gamut of investigations are negative and the final resort is to advise a laparotomy on the grounds that it may be a grumbling appendix, adhesions, glands or a possible carcinomatous condition. Sadly, the latter does sometimes occur but in a significant number of cases no abnormality is found.

Unexplained pain on the right side of the chest, for which X-rays are taken and no lung abnormality is discernible, may be labelled as pleurodynia or dry pleurisy. Neither of these words provides a sustainable diagnosis. The cause of the pain will almost invariably be found as a rheumatic patch located in the region of the pain distribution and the condition is quickly and efficiently treated with a sodium salicylate injection.

If the pain is on the left side, the question of angina then becomes dominant. The problem is aggravated because most people know about angina and, unless some rational explanation is available, fear and hence exaggeration of the symptoms develop. Cardiologists are consulted, and exhaustive investigations are undertaken. On the admission of cardiologists themselves, a diagnosis of angina is sometimes made without any true clinical or scientific evidence. Some have admitted that they are reluctant to give a complete clearance in case they are wrong and the patient later sustains a heart attack [19]. This is a good indication that they are so unsure of the clinical evidence that all the expensive scientific investigations which proclaim normality are not relied on.

Thus we have a considerable number of people who have no angina and no heart disease living in fear of having a heart attack!

Most of these cases can now be added to the numbers of pre-arthritics which are not recognised. Because no acceptable diagnosis has been made, some become classified as neurotic. It should not be too surprising that this happens. After all, have they not been fully and scientifically investigated by every relevant department? All specialists report, quite correctly, that there is no evidence of disease in their disciplines. Many of these patients are now treated with pain killers, sleeping tablets and tranquillisers. This hides their symptoms, clouds their thinking, and renders them submissive, thus removing the challenge for better diagnosis and treatment.

It is impossible to quote significant figures but the author has experience of a few patients treated in psychiatric hospitals.

It is from this great mass of patients that many seek help in paramedical areas. The greater the number that do this, the greater is the implicit challenge to medical failure.

The answer to most of these cases would have been found long before any investigations were undertaken, if only the physicians, surgeons and GPs were aware of the rheumatic patch. What we must all realise is that the rheumatic patch offers a new dimension in differential diagnosis based on the clinical history and physical findings in individual cases.

It is at this stage, and not before, that scientific aids should be used in either supporting or disproving the diagnosis. There is no short-cut in diagnosis. It has to be built up painstakingly on the pattern laid down by our predecessors. They painted clear pictures of disease from which this century's doctors can recognise, diagnose and apply modern scientific aids and treatments.

The latter cannot function successfully without that knowledge. A computer will provide a diagnosis of a doubtful case only from the data on diseases which have been fed into it. It therefore excludes all the problems which have so far been discussed, and these constitute about 80% of all suffering that afflicts mankind.

The rheumatic patch will explain a very high proportion of these cases and when they have been fed into the computer the number of unsolved 'diseases' will be dramatically reduced, as will the expense and workload which makes health services very costly without necessarily providing concomitant returns in increased health.

This chapter should be of special interest to all those doctors who have recently identified themselves as holistic in outlook. They wish to consider and treat the problems of each patient as a whole person, as against the established trends of specialisation which now appear to be the rigid infrastructure of medical education and practice.

I hope they will see from this chapter that every aspect of each individual patient has been taken into consideration in the planning of treatment. This is necessary because, as yet, there is no agreed medical understanding of what constitutes the life history of the rheumatic diseases, from their earliest symptoms to their final devastation of the human body, alive or dead. There can be little disagreement between us that my researches are based on the holistic conception and consequently the treatment has the same basis. In turn, these researches have been based entirely on the pattern which was laid down almost two centuries ago—when medical knowledge about disease was meagre. In those days, the doctors lived and worked amongst the patients—they collected the signs and symptoms, and gradually built up the coherent disease patterns we all know about and on which scientific medicine was based. As medical history unfolds we see how this method has given rise to cure and eradication of so many diseases. However, history seems now to have stopped unfolding where rheumatic disease is concerned.

It has been sectionalised or, if you prefer, specialised before its complete picture has been assembled. This in its turn has given rise to treatments which are not based on fundamental knowledge of the disease process, and can therefore never achieve a cure. Added to this failure is the damage done to the human body by the wide variety of poisonous drugs used for treatment [124]. This, I believe, is why the demand for holistic medicine is made. In my terms, it is saying do not treat patients with drugs until you understand the disease. It is better to use less harmful methods and to try to increase the natural resistance of the body. When the disease is fully understood, science will have a very much better chance of finding a real cure, as it has done in so many diseases which have been fully documented.

CHAPTER 8

The Skeleton—a New Concept

INTRODUCTION (W.W.F.)

From the evidence put forward up to this point it appears that the stability of the body cannot be ascribed to the bones, joints, ligaments and intervertebral discs alone. It is abundantly clear that the injection of relevant rheumatic patches restores stability and mobility while the arthritis remains unchanged in radiological terms. In rheumatoid arthritis where there is swelling, pain, weakness and restriction of movement in the fingers or wrists, immediate improvement takes place. This can best be described in the words of some patients: 'It feels as if all the joints have been oiled.'

A consideration of these quite remarkable results gave rise to the question, how can this be explained anatomically? The hypothesis put forward is that the role of the connective tissue in the maintenance of skeletal stability and joint function is much greater than generally accepted. This chapter describes the nature of connective tissue and then presents four different cases as a basis for discussion. These had not responded to any treatment previously tried elsewhere so that the results achieved might be considered good evidence in support of this line of thought.

CONNECTIVE TISSUE—WHAT IS IT? (D.L.J.F.)

Muscles, bones, tendons and other organs must be able to slide past each other if we are to be mobile. At the same time they must also be attached to each other, or we would fall apart. So there are two opposing imperatives, and the body's solution to the problem is connective tissue. It anchors the tissues and organs together, yet at the same time is stretchy enough to allow fairly free independent motion. Where greater degrees of mobility are required, the body provides a fluid-filled space, a joint or a bursa. Where less mobility and more strength are needed, the connective tissue coalesces and stiffens to form tendons, aponeuroses and ligaments. Joints and bursae are, from the histologist's viewpoint, simply clefts in the mesoderm; their inner surfaces are not lined with true epithelium and the fluid within them is simply a filtrate of plasma, with a little added glycosaminoglycan (hyaluronic acid) to provide viscosity [21].

If we were to remove the muscles, bones and visceral organs, we would be left with a semitranslucent 'ghost' of connective tissue, forming an interconnecting meshwork of hollow tubes and spaces of various sizes and shapes, rather like flexible sausage skins. Some would be roughly cigar shaped, two or three inches across and subdivided within by thinner sheets, to accommodate the muscles. Others would be long and thin—the sheaths of nerves and blood vessels. In some areas the tissues would condense and coalesce into tendons and ligaments. We would be able to see that every part of the edifice was in direct continuous contact with every other part, all being parts of a continuous whole. Without bones, of course, there would be no obvious shape, just a mound on the floor. But if we were to inflate the structure with air, a roughly human-shaped form would appear.

A mechanical stress applied to one part of this inflated structure would inevitably be felt in all other parts of the mass, as if we had filled a balloon with jelly, and were tapping one surface smartly with a spoon. To add the final realistic touches to this model we should have the inner surfaces of the jelly-filled balloon connected to each other within by long, thin ropes, criss-crossing the interior from side to side. By arranging these ropes so that radial ropes were all short, while longitudinal ropes were all long, we would change the shape of our balloon from a sphere to a sausage; more complex shapes could be devised

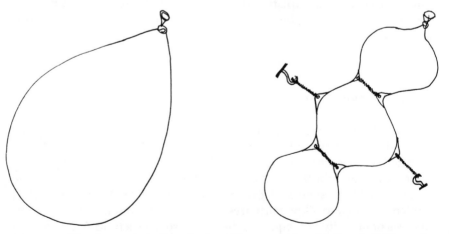

Figure 9   The shape of a balloon is altered by external and internal attachments.

simply by shortening or lengthening the ropes lying in any particular direction, or by tethering points of the outside of the balloon to nearby structures (figure 9).

This is actually pretty accurate as a picture of our connective tissues. The sac of our balloon is made of protein substances called collagen and elastin. The internal and external tethering ropes are made of collagen. The jelly filling the balloon is composed of carbohydrate molecules called glycosaminoglycans (GAGs). The inflation pressure of the balloon is provided by the GAGs, which have a huge capacity to absorb water, and hold it so that it cannot flow away. Collagen is a long and very tough protein molecule; it is very strong when pulled, but easily crumples if it is compressed. Elastin, as the name implies, provides stretchiness.

A reasonably functional body could be constructed in this way, without bones or joints, supported entirely by its own internal pressure. Many soft-bodied creatures, such as earthworms and jellyfish, do indeed function in just this way.

In real life, of course, we are also equipped with bones and joints, which means that our movements can be much faster and more precise, and also means that the inflation pressure of the balloon need not be so high as to make us impossibly stiff. The skeleton is attached to the connective tissues by the tendons, aponeuroses and ligaments noted before.

To understand the difference made by the skeleton we shall need to imagine a different type of structure. Consider a tent. The canvas is held aloft by the main tent poles, but these alone are not enough to create an edifice. For that, we need to stretch the canvas sideways and downwards using guy-ropes. The entire sheet of canvas is held under tension, but the tension is not uniform. It is concentrated at certain points—the apex of the tent, around the main poles, and the eyelets where the guy-ropes are attached. The manufacturer will often acknowledge this by reinforcing the points of attachment with leather or metal, since these points of concentrated tension are the points where tears will occur if the tension becomes too high.

If we now look back to our human-shaped, connective tissue 'ghost', draped over and attached to its skeleton like the canvas to its tent poles and guy-ropes, we can discern a number of attachments at which the tensions are concentrated. Indeed, if we look under the skin we will see that Nature has acknowledged this fact in the massive accumulations of dense fibrous connective tissue that we find there. One such point is the spine of the seventh cervical vertebra at the base of the neck, which carries the main burden of holding up the head (figure 10). Looked at from the back, the tension trajectories required to maintain an erect posture pass from the attachments of the trapezius muscles at the

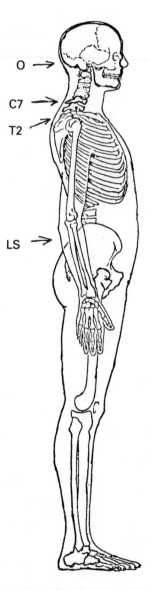

Figure 10   The centre of gravity of the skull lies in front of the spinal column in the neck, so gravity is always pulling the head forward and the head is held upright by tension between the occiput (O) and the seventh cervical spine (C7), as if by a rope attached at those two points. Similarly, the centre of gravity in the torso lies in front of the spine, so the natural fall of the body is forwards, and is resisted by ligaments and muscles pulling between approximately the second thoracic vertebra (T2) and the lumbo-sacral vertebrae (LS). By pulling T2 and LS together, the backward curve of the lumbar spine is maintained taut like a bow held by a bowstring.

occiput down to a roughly horizontal line across the back at the level of the tops of the scapulae, thence straight down the back to the dense fibrous tissue overlying the lumbo-sacral area and the sacro-iliac joints, which anchor the whole edifice (the tent-pegs).

We can now add muscles to the structure, to make movement possible and to complete our model man. The muscles take some of the tension away from the loose connective tissues, but they add to the tension concentrated on the tendons and aponeuroses.

We thus see that the concentrations of tension needed to maintain the erect human position are mainly dorsal, stretching from occiput to sacrum and being mainly concentrated around the base of the neck and the lumbo-sacral area. Rheumatic patches, as already noted, can occur anywhere in the body. However, the key rheumatic patches are mainly found dorsally, concentrated around the occiput, the base of the neck, and the lumbo-sacral area. It is these areas that must be treated before any others.

Tension and Compression—Ropes and Balloons

Ligaments and tendons, as noted above, are composed largely of collagen fibrils, arranged side by side into large rope-like molecules that are ideally adapted to their task of carrying considerable weights without stretching or breaking, but readily crumpling if compressed from end to end. However, even in a strong tissue such as tendon, there is always some of the other component, the GAGs that keep the tissue inflated with water. The ratio of collagen to GAG is higher in tendon, and lower in cartilage and loose ariolar tissue, but these two basic components are always present [22].

GAGs are long carbohydrate molecules consisting of chains of monosaccharides (sugars), usually of two alternating types. Individual GAGs have their own names: chondroitin sulphate, dermatan sulphate and keratan sulphate. As is evident from the names, all carry multiple sulphate groups, which confer a net negative electric charge on the molecule which in turn attracts small positively charged ions (sodium, potassium, calcium, etc.). Each GAG molecule is therefore normally surrounded by an attendant cloud of positive ions, which increase the osmolarity of the tissue and serve to attract and hold water molecules (the Donnan effect) [23, 24].

The GAG chains are normally attached to protein 'backbone' chains, like the bristles of a bottle-brush, to form larger aggregates called proteoglycans, and the proteoglycans are themselves attached to enormously long chains of another GAG, hyaluronic acid (enormously long in molecular terms, that is). Each proteoglycan–hyaluronic acid molecule, although huge in molecular terms, is still just one molecule in its physical behaviour. Although its molecular weight is around 50 million daltons, it contributes exactly the same osmotic effect as a sodium ion of 23 daltons. To all intents and purposes, therefore, the fluid-holding properties of connective tissue are entirely controlled by the small positive ions, and these in turn are controlled by the sulphation of the GAGs as well as by the electrical charge on the tissue (see below).

Connective tissues of various types are therefore composite materials. Like fibreglass or reinforced concrete, connective tissues consist of a 'fluid' matrix penetrated by and attached onto fibres. Composite materials have a physics all of their own, and all share certain properties. One of these characteristics is that if a composite is stretched from top to bottom or from side to side, and if within that composite there is a small piece of stiffer material, the stress trajectories become concentrated into the stiffer patch (figure 12) [25].

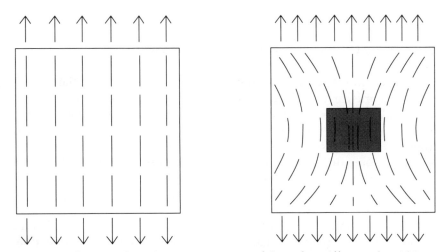

Figure 11   Stress trajectories are concentrated into the stiffer patch within a composite material.

This will inevitably occur if a connective tissue contains a rheumatic patch, since these are always stiffer than the surrounding tissue (that is how they can be palpated). Concentrations of tension, as noted above when considering the behaviour of tent canvas, can lead to tears and other mechanical damage, so that a composite material can paradoxically be weakened by the insertion of a stronger piece [25].

Another fascinating property of connective tissue is **piezoelectricity**: the generation of small electrical charges across the material when it is stretched or otherwise deformed (the same principle, in reverse, is used in quartz watches). The piezoelectricity of connective tissue is mainly due to the collagen within it, and the tissue does not have to be alive. Even dead collagen is piezoelectric [25].

The metabolism of cells when alive is, however, strongly influenced by ambient electric fields [26], so when a piezoelectric potential is set up within a connective tissue by stretching it, one would expect the cells of that tissue to respond with greater or lesser metabolic rates. Another point about piezoelectricity is that it provides a primitive but very fast and sensitive communication network within connective tissues: no part of a connective tissue structure can escape knowing when another part of the structure is under stress, and this communication is completely independent of the nervous system. It does not require nerves or even life.

CASE STUDIES (W.W.F.)

Case 1

Patient: T.J.S. (female), 17½ years
First consultation: August 27, 1982

Three years of constant ache in the left back and hip with severe pain on weight bearing. The hip feels as if it is dislocated and she has to click it back into position before she can attempt to rise from a sitting position, which is difficult and painful.

She takes up to six paracetamols and three Distalgesics every day to control the pain.

Examination
Examination confirmed the marked loss of mobility due to severe pain. Many areas of tenderness (rheumatic patches) were found in the left lumbar and gluteal areas.

Treatment
Injection of a rheumatic patch in the lumbar area produced an immediate response. For the first time in over a year she was able to rise from the chair and sit down again with almost no pain or effort. Walking capacity greatly improved.

From October 27, 1982, to August 11, 1983, 14 treatments were given. She now walks normally, rarely has pain, her hip does not 'dislocate' and she needs no analgesics. The X-ray is presented in figure 12.

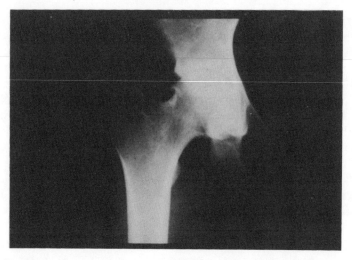

Figure 12   X-ray showing arthritis of the right hip.

Case 2

Patient: T.S. (male), 28 years
First consultation: March 25, 1982

Since 1980 he complained of severe pain night and day in the right leg from the lower back to below the knee. In order to walk at all he has to flex his trunk and bend the knee.

History
December 1978: motor accident. Fracture of right acetabulum. Four weeks traction followed by operation and insertion of two screws into acetabulum. Made good progress with no limp or pain.

January 1979: X-ray shows screws and normal head of femur. April 1979: discarded calliper, continued free of disability until September 1980, when his present symptoms began.

The condition continued to deteriorate with the severe pain moving to all parts of the leg whether standing, sitting or lying down. X-ray in January 1982 showed collapse of femoral head.

Examination
Examination confirmed wasting to right thigh and leg with 1½ inch shortening. Severe limitation of movement due to pain. There were widespread areas of tenderness in dorsal area and in the leg (rheumatic patches).

Treatment
Injection of the patches with sodium salicylate was begun. There was an immediate response—he was able to unflex his body to an upright position and was able to walk with less pain. Further treatments were given from May 13, 1982, to May 6, 1983, during which time the condition has greatly improved.

The X-ray is presented in figure 13.

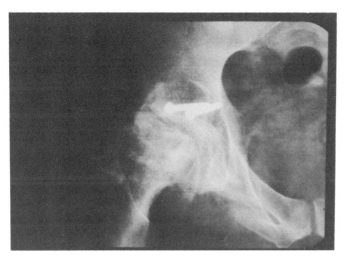

Figure 13 X-ray showing ischaemic necrosis at the head of the right femur.

Case 3

Patient: A.R. (female), 92 years
First consultation: June 17, 1983

Complains of very severe and persistent pain in right leg and is unable to walk on it. She also has constant pain in lower dorsal and lumbar area spreading to right groin. Has been prescribed pain killers and anti-rheumatic drugs.

In April 1983, investigated in hospital for severe flare-up of condition. X-ray showed gross arthritis and collapse of lumbar vertebra. Hips appeared normal.

Examination
Examination confirmed that patient was unable to hold her back straight because of pain and loss of power. She was wearing a corset to support

her back. Great difficulty in walking. There were many areas of tenderness on the right trunk (rheumatic patches).

Treatment
Injection of sodium salicylate into patch extending from level dorsal 9 to lumbar 4 reduced the back pain considerably. She was then able to hold her body erect and walking became marginally easier.

June 26: maintained much of the improvement except groin pain. Further injections given in lumbar area which were followed by more improvement in groin pain and walking.

August: three treatments each producing further improvement.

She has remained completely free from back pain, has abandoned the corset and is able to sit normally in a chair.

The X-ray is presented in figure 14.

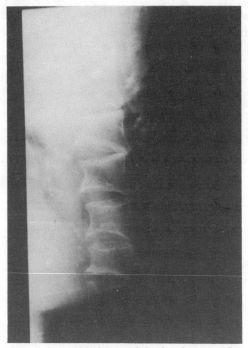

Figure 14   X-ray showing osteoarthritis of the lumbar vertebrae.

Case 4

Patient: S.S. (male), 52 years
First consultation: November 5, 1981

He complained of persistent pain in the neck for seven years with marked limitation of movement. The symptoms started 12 years ago but were intermittent and gradually becoming more frequent and persistent.

History
He had a racing car accident about two years before the symptoms began. He does not recall any adverse effect immediately after the accident.

August 1979: a neurologist reported a spastic tetraparesis, with increased tendon jerks in all four limbs, clonus at both ankles and extensor plantar responses. There is a suggestion of slight relative reduction of the supinator jerk on the left side, by comparison with the other jerks, but finger jerks are brisk on both sides and Hofman's sign is positive. There is slight reduction of vibration sense at the ankles.

November 9, 1979: myelogram showed extensive obliteration of the root pouches C3/4, 4/5, 5/6 on both sides with some compression of the cord at C4/5 and 5/6 levels (see figure 15). He was subsequently advised that an operation on the cervical vertebrae was the only option for him.

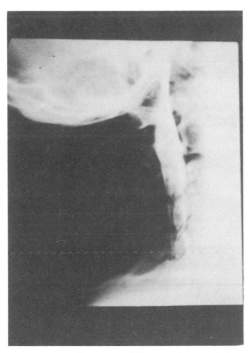

Figure 15   X-ray showing myelogram of the cervical vertebrae.

Examination
Examination confirmed almost total lack of movement of the neck and

very tender areas in the connective tissue of the posterior aspect of the neck.

Treatment

A rheumatic patch in the neck was injected. Immediate result, the pain lessened considerably and he was able to move his neck remarkably freely.

He has had six further treatments up to July 25, 1983, mostly for very slight symptoms.

All the abnormal reflexes had returned to normal with the exception of very slight clonus of the right ankle.

The X-ray is presented in figure 15.

Because the pain, reflexes and neck movement were so much better it did not seem justifiable to submit him to another myelogram.

DISCUSSION   (W.W.F.)

Cases 1 and 2 indicate that the strength and power of the connective tissue when the rheumatic patches are treated is sufficient to improve stability of the hip in one case of osteoarthritis and, in the other, when the head of the femur had collapsed.

Case 3 shows that after treatment of the rheumatic patches the connective tissue was able to hold the spinal column in an upright position, even though the dorsal and lumbar vertebrae were grossly deformed by arthritis.

Case 4 indicates that pressure on the spinal cord due to arthritis in the cervical vertebrae could be reduced by the power of the connective tissue, when the inflammation has been improved. It is probably achieved because this tissue can now hold the vertebrae in their correct position, thus preventing pressure on the cord. This case has been included because it demonstrates in the most positive way the effect on the cervical vertebrae of removing the inflammation from the rheumatic patch. It is hoped that these detailed clinical findings will help you to accept the idea of the common identity of pathology in any part of the vertebral column.

To explain the mechanism by which the rheumatic patch first causes pain and disability, and later determines the onset of arthritis in the vertebra, we must first identify the basic relationship between the connective tissue with the bones and joints in the maintenance of skeletal integrity.

For an analogy, let us consider the earthworm. It consists of a tube of longitudinal and circular muscles containing reproductive organs, a brain and five 'hearts'. All are held together by connective tissue. The movements of the worm are elementary. It can go forward by contracting the circular muscles and elongating the longitudinal muscles in its anterior segments, forming a spear-like head, and at the same time the muscles at the rear end must do exactly the opposite in order to form a squat stub end which acts as the fulcrum so that it can propel itself forward. It cannot turn sideways at all and cannot go backwards except by anchoring its rear segment to the earth and propelling itself backwards to the fulcrum of the fixed point.

Let us assume the worm needs to turn its anterior half to the right or left. It would need to develop a hardened piece of connective tissue in mid-line from which the anterior half could launch itself in the required direction—this would be the fulcrum. The connective tissue is thus firmly attached to the fulcrum, closely invests all the muscles and together they form a unit of movement within the original framework of the worm. The formation of further units will enable more varieties of movement until we finally reach the position of mankind, where the separation of hardened areas (bones) become necessary and so joints are formed.

The human foetus shows this development of bone structure within the collagen tissue, thus confirming the interdependence of both structures but within the original function of the connective tissue.

Throughout all this development the connective tissue is the constant factor, thickening and thinning, forming relative amounts of elastin and collagen fibres as the need arises, so as always to maintain its integrated control of the locomotor system.

It is at this point that we must change our concept that the tissue is 'connective', just holding bones or joints together in a passive way. This tissue envelops the whole locomotor system—the bones, joints, muscles and tendons—and is loosely connected by strands to the skin. The tissue must exert some control over these components in order to achieve the concerted rhythmic action of the muscles which produces the enormous variety of movement available to the body.

The tensile strength of tendon is about 10 000 times greater than muscle [20]. When the muscle contracts in order that its tendon can exert a force on the bones or joints to which it is attached, it would be torn to shreds were it not for the collagen fibres which are strong enough to take the strain and thus to protect the actual muscle fibres.

What is suggested is that the real skeleton is the connective tissue, from which the bones and joints have developed later in order to give shape (e.g. the thorax), varieties of movement (e.g. the wrists) and the fulcra, from which the connective tissue can exert its pull (e.g. the vertebrae).

The bones and joints are passive structures which are manipulated by the muscles and tendons and held in any required position, controlled and protected by the all-pervading connective tissue.

How else would it be possible to achieve the remarkable contortions of the spine by a gymnast, where one part of the dorsal spine is held rigid as solid bone, while the next segment is flexing and in a split second the flexing can be moved to the previously solid portion? Just as remarkable is the ability of a ballet dancer to stand poised on the toes of one foot. Given that no movement can take place without the participation of the connective tissue, it now becomes understandable that a rheumatic patch will cause pain and restriction of movement when the affected area is required to function. The severity of the symptoms will depend on the extent of the rheumatic patch and bears no relationship whatever to the X-ray picture of arthritis in the vertebra: the most obvious form of low back pain is acute lumbago, which occurs at almost any age from second to sixth decade; in all the younger groups there is no evidence of lumbar arthritis and it is only as they get older that a gradual development of osteoarthritis can be noted.

In those cases where injury, strain or sprain are considered to be the cause of the backache the question must be asked, why do some clear up quickly when others persist for months or even years? The answer is to be found by clinical examination, when the presence of rheumatic patches aggravated by the injury will be found, and their treatment immediately improves or abolishes the symptoms.

There is another aspect to this problem which can be understood only if the significance of the rheumatic patch is appreciated. Many people suddenly and quite unexpectedly develop a back problem while doing some work in the garden, e.g. digging or weeding, or in the home, e.g. moving some furniture or climbing stairs, or even bending to put shoes on.

The identical problem is common in all forms of sport, where it is even more pertinent to consider that, in the case of professionals, all these activities have been done throughout their lives, so why should a simple repetition in one particular instance give rise to pain and disability?

Patients have been closely questioned about these incidents and it is quite clear the pain sometimes comes on (a) just as they were about to bend, (b) in the act of bending or (c) some time after the activity ceased. In all these cases patients do not make these distinctions, so that the activity is blamed for the symptom and is accepted by them and the doctor.

It is quite startling to find that terms such as sprain, pulled muscle, strained tendon or torn ligament are still represented, without a shred of clinical evidence, to be the cause of the symptoms. The real pathology, where the so-called injury is spurious, is a sudden reactivation of an old rheumatic patch or the formation of a new one.

Because the patches are inflammatory in nature their onset can almost always be related to a recent 'cold' or more realistically a sore throat and upper respiratory infection, some generalised aching such as influenza, lack of energy and depression [3, 7].

At the time of their occurrence, unless they are very severe, they are ignored because most people do not like 'making a fuss' and want to get on with their activities. They are never consciously associated with the 'injury' which soon follows and are totally forgotten.

It is the recurrence of these episodes during the lifetime of the individual which, by gradually damaging more and more of the connective tissue, affects the integrity of the locomotor system. Where the lower back is concerned, bending and straightening become less easy, stiffness becomes more marked and balancing of the body becomes more hazardous, for example when putting on trousers or walking on uneven surfaces or up and down stairs.

All these facts are part of the clinical story of the chronic rheumatic diseases which I have already detailed and now wish to emphasise.

The lipping of the vertebrae, which does not always follow a precise pattern, can now be explained by the unequal forces being exerted on them because part of the connective tissue affected by the rheumatic patch is unable to function normally. In addition, the patient learns how to avoid or at least to minimise the pain by adjusting the posture and so throwing further strain on relatively healthy connective tissue, thus increasing the unequal pull on the vertebral edges. Equally it can explain the variations in the erosions in the acetabulum and head of the femur.

In this sequence of events we can see how an inflamed pathology in the connective tissue can initiate a non-inflammatory arthritis in the lumbar vertebra.

The logic of this is that arthritis of the spine is the end-result of a pathology in the connective tissue and cannot be the cause of the original pain and disability.

Failure to solve the problem of arthritis must be due in part to the almost universal acceptance of bone and joint pathology demonstrable by X-ray as a starting point of the disability and its investigation. This is no less fallacious than attributing locomotor ataxia to the pathology in the spinal cord, when the original cause was a chancre contracted many years ago.

In its turn the development of arthritis can be much better understood with the realisation that the rheumatic patch precedes it, and is the initial and main cause of the symptoms.

What remains to be explained is, how does the local treatment of a rheumatic patch in the superficial fascia give rise to such dramatic and instant improvement in mobility to the related part of the body? In the fields of anatomy and biomechanics there is no change in the view that the deep fascia is an important factor in locomotion but that the superficial fascia has no significant role to play. The above results quite obviously suggest that some vital knowledge is missing, which could demonstrate that the superficial fascia, far from being insignificant, has a major role in skeletal integrity.

The theory of piezoelectricity discussed earlier by Dr. Freed (pp. 94–95) offers an acceptable explanation of the dramatic results of treating a rheumatic patch over the lower cervical and upper dorsal area, which improves the condition of the arms and hands.

Further research into these phenomena should eventually provide an unequivocal explanation. When this is achieved, it must radically alter much present-day medical thinking. This should give rise to new and simpler methods of dealing with skeletal problems such as lordosis and kyphosis, and all the deformities which are wrongly ascribed to the arthritides.

CHAPTER 9

The Way Forward (W.W.F.)

The discovery of the rheumatic patch brought a real understanding of the basic pathology in these diseases. It is the undeniable link and the common factor, not only of the chronic rheumatic diseases, but of all problems which, at present, are not recognised or understood as being rheumatic in origin.

All my work has been based on the teachings of orthodox medicine. Paradoxically, because scientific medicine has often developed so rapidly as to leave behind the orthodox basic concepts of the great clinicians of the past, it is me who is often accused of being unorthodox!

I do not claim that these methods represent a cure for any form of arthritis. This can never be achieved until the causative agent has been identified.

My researches have shown that the onset of most arthritic disease is not in the joints—that comes much later—but in the superficial connective tissue. It does not seem unreasonable to me to suggest that is why the widespread investigation of the joints for so many years has failed to offer any prospect of finding a cause or cure.

It is possible that, where allergic and immunological problems are the dominant factors in any particular cases, they can be greatly improved or even cured if treatment so alters the physiology of the body that it is able to overcome the pathological agent, even if it has not been identified. Where this is achieved, the rheumatic patches of long standing will still need to be treated in order to restore maximum movement and minimum pain. In the meantime, the methods of treatment outlined in this book will most certainly reduce the ravages of the disease, so that when it eventually burns out, as in rheumatoid arthritis, the patient will have very much less disability and deformity than is now so common. This would reduce the need for surgical intervention and so materially help in the reduction and expense of these procedures.

More importantly, the continued study of the rheumatic patch, both in treatment and scientific investigation, may well produce the answer we all want—the pathogen which starts the disease process.

Dr. Freed's excellent analysis of the problems in the immune system suggests to me that it is not vital to differentiate between the possibility of a foreign invader such as a virus and an ingested protein such as a lectin. At this point it would not be inappropriate to consider homeopathic treatment.

The basic concept, as I understand, is that most symptoms are caused by poisons which may be ingested, imbibed or inhaled. By the study of their toxic effects, it is possible to relate the patient's symptoms to the likeliest poisons.

The treatment is based on the dictum that like cures like. This means that minute amounts of the suspected poisons are given to the patient, so that the body learns to identify and overcome them. It is surely a form of immunisation which should be totally acceptable to orthodox medicine, and runs parallel with a possible virus or lectin. I would like to state here that when I worked with Mr. W. E. Tucker, the orthopaedic surgeon at the Royal London Homeopathic Hospital, the hospital medical committee allowed me to use the diphtheroid vaccine on the patients I treated because they accepted that such treatment was in accordance with their precepts.

What we need to do is to pursue these closely related phenomena in relation to the superficial connective tissue precisely because they precede joint pathology.

The response to treatment of the rheumatic patch with local anaesthetic or sodium salicylate solution is so immediate and dramatic in over 80% of cases that there can be little doubt about the key position it holds in the early development of rheumatic pathology. This in its turn has given rise to the concept that the function of the normal superficial connective tissue has a much greater role than has so far been realised in the maintenance of skeletal integrity.

Together with these concepts there is the lateral thinking in 1947 which gave rise to the use of Corynebacteria as a method of combating the infective agent (virus) in these diseases. I know that the evidence produced then is quite insufficient to be accepted by modern standards. For that matter, I did not think it was sufficient even in 1950. My aim in publishing the paper was to interest the scientific and research departments of hospitals to pursue these ideas. There were no such facilities available to me. It took 30 years for scientists to confirm the logical assumptions made then, without their being aware of my publications in 1950. On that basis, clinical and scientific corroboration of the rheumatic patch is just about due, while the true function of the superficial connective tissue might take another 10–20 years.

Over the last three decades various spokespersons for rheumatology have publicly stated that a solution of the arthritis problem could be hoped for in 5 years. Because my studies taught me the relative unimportance of the actual joint disease, I was convinced their hopes would not be sustained. Nowadays, there are few in the profession who believe that continuing research on the old lines is ever likely to succeed. Hence the increasing adoption of para-medical practices, e.g. acupuncture, osteopathy or manipulative techniques, together with the endless supply of new drugs.

Paradoxically, because of the first perceptible interest in my lines of research, I am hopeful that a solution will be found within five years. In the meantime, my main concern is to disseminate the knowledge of the rheumatic patch throughout the profession because it has two important roles to fulfil.

First, it not only establishes a relationship between different types of arthritis, but also signposts the clinical development of the disease process from childhood to old age. Only in this way will the rheumatic story be as complete as those for all the other diseases such as influenza, poliomyelitis, diphtheria, measles, bacterial pneumonia and tuberculosis which are now successfully treated or controlled.

The second reason is that it offers a simple explanation of all those problems enumerated in a previous chapter on differential diagnosis. If general practitioners knew about the rheumatic patch, it would resolve so many problems which they now refer to hospitals where they are investigated for diseases that might be and never turn out to be. What an appalling waste of time, money and resources, with no resolution of the patient's problem. How much more satisfying for the GP to make the right diagnosis by a simple physical examination which costs nothing but a few minutes in time, and then to relieve the symptoms by an equally simple injection.

This would apply to at least 50% of all such cases even in relatively inexperienced hands. With increasing experience, the percentage would climb to 70%–80% while some of the remainder could be recognised as an active state of some of the more serious developments of rheumatoid arthritis, lupus erythematosis or polymyalgia.

If the truth of these findings is accepted, then it is doubly important that it should be taught to all medical students so that its significance is known to potential physicians and surgeons in any discipline where the rheumatic patch can mimic the disease in which they specialise. There will then be no difficulty in separating them from those diseases without having to pursue expensive investigations.

In the orthopaedic field many of the spinal fusion operations will become superfluous, while the ease with which kyphosis and lordosis can be improved should remove the constant sight of elderly people with bent back and walking sticks on our pavements.

Being fully conversant with medical teaching and, hence, thinking, over the last six decades, I understand the incredulity these facts will arouse. Wherever I have demonstrated or lectured, from the Scripps Clinic and Research Foundation in California in 1981, to the International Rheumatic Congress in Jerusalem in November 1986, the enthusiasm and interest has been more than encouraging.

In 1983, after a seminar at Hope Hospital, Salford, part of the Rheumatic Unit of Manchester University, arrangements were made to institute clinical trials which never materialised.

In 1984, successful clinical demonstrations on four consecutive weeks were made at the Eastbourne General Hospital, England. Efforts by Dr. Jan Wojtulewski, Head of the Department of Rheumatology, and myself to set up clinical trials were thwarted by the difficulties of financing and organising the experiment.

In 1986, a lecture at the Kennedy Institute gave rise to a tentative arrangement to institute limited trials at Charing Cross Hospital. Professor Maini, Head of both the Kennedy Institute and the Rheumatic Department of West London Hospital, was most supportive but it was still not possible to implement the agreed procedure. Further efforts by Professor Maini are now in progress to establish trials at the West London Hospital.

In the meantime, I would make the following suggestions for an immediate test of my claims. Selection should be made of:

1. (a) A number of cases of osteoarthritis of the hip who are waiting for surgery.
   (b) An equal number of rheumatoid arthritis cases whose hands are becoming weak, painful and deformed.
   (c) An equal number of chronic backache cases.
2. Any type of rheumatic cases presenting at an outpatient session or in a group practice. The only proviso I would make is that no patient on oral steroid therapy be accepted for the trial.

They need be treated in the first place only with local anaesthetic, to demonstrate the first and immediate signs of improvement.

Such investigations do not require reference to any ethical committee and it should be enough to convince any observer of the link between three 'diseases' which are considered to be entirely unrelated by the orthodox establishment in the Western world.

I must perforce leave out the Eastern bloc because, as indicated earlier in the text, a form of my treatment is nationally available in Bulgaria. The ideas, the facts and the evidence submitted in these pages should not be dismissed because they appear to conflict with present-day views. They are merely inserting clinical facts in the natural history of the chronic rheumatic diseases.

May I quote from an English translation of a preface by Dr. Marcos

Cots, Orthopaedic Surgeon, Barcelona Hospital, Spain, who wrote the preface to the Spanish edition of my book *Arthritis—Is Your Suffering Really Necessary?*

'Personally, as an orthopaedic surgeon, I have to say that the experiences of Dr. Fox [have] awakened my total interest. You can agree or disagree with his methods but nobody can deny his very good results and on many occasions positively spectacular results. And no human being has the right to deny the propagation of his methods. Having read his work, I feel we owe Dr. Fox a vote of confidence and [should] treat his work with the same attention we gave to the teachings of our old professors when we were simple students.'

Have not the patients suffered long enough? Has not the medical profession travailed long enough to make us doubt the value of the lines of treatment and research in the last 40 years? Should we not now tread the old path which proceeds directly from pure clinical findings which was crowned with so much success in the last four decades?

I believe the time has surely arrived when the claims made here should be challenged and investigated. Only in this way can reality and truth be tested. That is all I have ever asked.

References

[1] Scott, D. L., Symmons, D. P. M., Coulton, B. L., and Popert, A. J. (1987). Long-term outcome of treating rheumatoid arthritis: results after 20 years. *Lancet*, **i**, 1108–1111.

[2] Bjarnasson, I., Zanelli, G., Prouse, P., Smethurst, P., Smith, T., Levi, S., Gumpel, M. J., and Levi, A. J. (1987). Blood and protein loss via small-intestinal inflammation induced by non-steroidal anti-inflammatory drugs. *Lancet*, **ii**, 711–714.

[3] Fox, W. W. (1950). A clinical study of the chronic rheumatic diseases. *J. Rheum.* (January).

[4] Tsomkov, A. (1986). Arthrosis is curable. *Bulg. Trade J.*, No. 3 (May–June).

[5] Bitnum, S. (1987). Hip pain in children. *Prog. Rheumatol.*, **3**, 252–258.

[6] Fox, W. W. (1966). A new approach to the medical treatment of osteoarthritis of the hip. *Br. J. Clin. Pract.*, **20** (12).

[7] Fox, W. W. (1975). *Arthritis and Allied Conditions*, Dr. William W. Fox, London.

[8] Douthwaite, E. H. (1948). *Practitioner*, **161**, 153.

[9] Decker, J. L., and Glossary Subcommittee of the ARA Committee on Rheumatologic Practice. (1983). American Rheumatism Association nomenclature and classification of arthritis and rheumatism.

[10] Broder, I., Baumal, R., Gordon D., and Bell, D. (1969). Histamine-releasing activity of rheumatoid and non-rheumatoid serum and synovial fluid. *Ann. NY Acad. Sci.*, **168**, 126–139.

[11] Fox, W. W. (1981). *Arthritis — Is Your Suffering Really Necessary?*, Robert Hale, London.

[12] Fox, W. W. (1987). The rheumatic patch. *Progress in Rheumatology*, Vol. III, *The Fourth International Seminar on the Treatment of Rheumatic Disease*, Golda Medical Centre, Petah-Tiqva, pp. 242–245.

[13] Eastoe, J. E., and Courts, A. (1963). *Practical Analytical Methods for Connective Tissue Proteins*, E. & F. N. Spon, London.

[14] Warter, P. J., Davis, D. A., and Horoschak, S. (1947). *J. Med. Soc. NJ*, **44**, 441.

[15] Bacon, T. H., De Vere-Tyndall, A., Tyrrell, D. A. J., Denman, A. M., and Ansell, B. M. (1983). Interferon system in patients with systemic juvenile chronic arthritis. *In vivo* and *in vitro* studies. *Clin. Exp. Immunol.*, **54**, 23–30.

[16] Werner, G. H. (1979). *Pharm. Ther. J.*, **16**, 235.

[17] Zuraw, B. L., O'Hair, C. H., Vaughan, J. H., Mathison, D. A., Curd, J. C., and Katz, D. H. (1981). Immunoglobulin E — rheumatoid factor in the serum of patients with rheumatoid arthritis, asthma and other diseases. *J. Clin. Invest.*, **68** (December), 1610–1613.

[18] HMSO (1987). *UK Government Report. Costs and Benefits of Pharmaceutical Research*, HMSO, London.

[19] Pappworth, M. H. (1978). Diagnosing angina pectoris. *World Med.* (May 17).

[20] Gordon, A. H., Martin, A. J. P., and Gynge, R. L. M. (1943). *Biochem. J.*, **37**, 79.

[21] Fassbender, H. G. (1975). *The Pathology of Rheumatic Diseases*, Springer, Berlin.

[22] Hukins, D. W. L., and Aspden, R. M. (1985). Composition and properties of connective tissues. *Trends Biochem. Sci.*, **10**, 260–264.

[23] Myers, E. R., Armstrong, C. G., and Mow, V. C. (1984). Swelling pressure and collagen tension. In Hukins, D. W. L. (ed.), *Connective Tissue Matrix*, Macmillan, Basingstoke, pp. 161–186.

[24] Bayliss, M. T. (1984). Proteoglycans: structure and molecular organisation in cartilage. In Hukins, D. W. L. (ed.), *Connective Tissue Matrix*, Macmillan, Basingstoke, pp. 55–88.

[25] Hukins, D. W. L. (1982). Biomechanical properties of collagen. In Weiss, J. B., and Jayson, M. I. V. (eds.), *Collagen in Health and Disease*, Churchill Livingstone, Edinburgh, pp. 49–72.

[26] Polk, C., and Postow, E. (eds.) (1986). *CRC Handbook of Biological Effects of Electromagnetic Fields*, CRC Press, Boca Raton, FL.

[27] Sokoloff, L. (1984). Animal models of rheumatoid arthritis. In Richter, G. W., and Epstein, M. A. (eds.), *International Review of Experimental Pathology*, Vol. 26, Academic Press, Orlando, FL, pp. 107–145.

[28] Phillips, P. E., and Christian, C. L. (1982). Infectious agents in chronic rheumatic disease. In McCarty, D. J. (ed.), *Arthritis and Allied Conditions, a Textbook of Rheumatology*, Lea and Febiger, Philadelphia, PA, pp. 431–449.

[29] Partsch, G., Gialamas, J., Adamiker, D., Höger, H., Neumüller, J., and Eberl, R. (1986). Induction of arthritic processes by synovial fluids of rheumatoid arthritis patients in long-term experiments with mice. *Int. J. Tissue React.*, **8**, 303–307.

[30] Fassbender, H. G. (1975). *The Pathology of Rheumatic Diseases*, Springer, Berlin, pp. 79 *et seq.*

[31] Cailliet, R. (1983). Foreword. In Travell, J. G., and Simons, D. G. (eds.), *Myofascial Pain and Dysfunction: the Trigger Point Manual*, Williams & Wilkins, Baltimore, MD, p. xi.

[32] Reinert, O. C. (1976). *Chiropractic Procedure and Practice*, Marian Press, Florissant, MO, pp. 264 *et seq.*

[33] Mann, F. (1971). *Acupuncture: the Ancient Chinese Art of Healing*, Heinemann, London, pp. 28–30.

[34] Travell, J. G., and Simons, D. G., (eds.) (1983). *Myofascial Pain and Dysfunction: the Trigger Point Manual*, Williams & Wilkins, Baltimore, MD, pp. 2–18.

[35] Sinclair, D. C. (1949). The remote reference of pain aroused in the skin. *Brain*, **72**, 364–372.

[36] Ongley, M. J., Klein, R. G., Dorman, T. A., Eek, B. C., and Hubert, L. J. (1987). A new approach to the treatment of chronic low back pain. *Lancet*, **ii**, 143–146.

[37] Rush, P. J., Shore, A., Inman, R., Gold, R., Jadavji, T., and Laski, B. (1986). Arthritis associated with *Haemophilus influenzae* meningitis; septic or reactive? *J. Pediatr.*, **109**, 412–415.

[38] Cooper, C., Muhlemann, M., Wright, D. J. M., Hutchinson, C. A., Armstrong, R., and Maini, R. N. (1987). Arthritis as manifestation of Lyme disease in England. *Lancet*, **i**, 1313–1314.

[39] Goodman-Gilman, A., Goodman, L. S., Gilman, A., Mayer, S. E., and Melmon, K. L. (eds.) (1980). *Goodman and Gilman's The Pharmacological Basis of Therapeutics*, Macmillan, New York, pp. 688–698.

[40] Stuart, J. M., Townes, A. S., and Kang, A. H. (1984). Collagen autoimmune arthritis. *Ann. Rev. Immunol.*, **2**, 199–218.

[41] Frost, F. A., Jessen, B., and Siggard-Andersen, J. (1980). A controlled double-blind comparison of mepivacaine injection versus saline injection for myofascial pain. *Lancet*, **i**, 499–504.

[42] Campbell, S. M., Clark, S., Tindall, E. A., Forehand, M. E., and Bennett, R. M. (1983). Clinical characteristics of fibrositis I: a 'blinded' controlled study of symptoms and tender points. *Arthritis Rheum.*, **26**, 817–824.

[43] Berek, J. S., Knapp, R. C., Hacker, N. F., Lichtenstein, A., Jung, T., Spina, C., Obrist, R., Griffiths, C. T., Berkowitz, R. S., Parker, L., Zighelboim, J., and Bast, R. C. (1985). Intraperitoneal immunotherapy of epithelial ovarian carcinoma with *Corynebacterium parvum*. *Am. J. Obstet. Gynecol.*, **152**, 1003–1010.

[44] Mastroeni, P., Bizzini, B., Bonina, L., *et al.* (1985). The restoration of impaired macrophage functions using as immunomodulator the *Corynebacterium granulosum*-derived P40 fraction. *Immunopharmacology*, **10**, 27–34.

[45] Iannello, D., Bonina, L., Merendino, R. A., *et al.* (1985). Evaluation of *Corynebacterium granulosum* derived P40 fraction: effects on macrophage anti-herpes simplex virus type I functions. *Antiviral Res.*, *Suppl. 1*, 167–171.

[46] Freed, D. L. J. (1982). The immunology of allergy. In Rees, A., and Purcell, H. (eds.), *Disease and the Environment*, Wiley, Chichester.

[47] Gupta, S., and Good, R. A. (eds.) (1979). *Cellular, Molecular and Clinical Aspects of Allergic Disorders*, Comprehensive Immunology, Vol. 6, Plenum, New York.

[48] Freed, D. L. J., Buckley, C. H., Tsivion, Y., Sharon, N., and Katz, D. (1983). Non-allergenic haemolysins in grass pollens and housedust mites. *Allergy*, **38**, 477–486.

[49] Silverstone, G. A. (1985). Possible sources of food toxicants. In Seely, S., Freed, D. L. J., Silverstone, G. A., and Rippere, V. (eds.), *Diet Related Diseases: The Modern Epidemic*, Croom Helm, London, pp. 40–118.

[50] Eaton, K. K. (1982). The incidence of allergy . . . has it changed? *Clin. Allergy*, **12**, 107–110.

[51] Ward, A. G., and Courts, A. (eds.) (1977). *The Science and Technology of Gelatin*, Academic Press, London.

[52] Steven, F. S. (1967). The effect of chelating agents on collagen interfibrillar matrix interactions in connective tissue. *Biochim. Biophys. Acta*, **140**, 522–528.

[53] Courts, A. (1980). Properties and uses of gelatin. In Grant, R. A. (ed.), *Applied Protein Chemistry*, Applied Science Publishers, Barking, pp. 14–18.

[54] Courts, A. (1961). Structural changes in collagen II: enhanced solubility of bovine collagen: reactions with hydrogen peroxide and some properties of soluble eucollagen. *Biochem. J.*, **81**, 356–364.

[55] Brauer, R., Thoss, K., Henzgen, S., and Waldmann, G. (1985). Lectin-induced arthritis of rabbit as a model of rheumatoid arthritis. In Bøg-Hansen, T. C., and Breborowicz, J. (eds.), *Lectins: Biology, Biochemistry, Clinical Biochemistry*, Vol. 4, de Gruyter, Berlin, pp. 28–38.

[56] Parke, A. C., and Hughes, G. R. V. (1981). Rheumatoid arthritis and food; a case study. *Br. Med. J.*, **282**, 2027–2029.

[57] Pinals, R. S. (1986). Arthritis associated with gluten-sensitive enteropathy. *J. Rheumatol.*, **13**, 201–204.

[58] Mäki, M., Hällström, O., Verronen, P., Reunala, T., Lähdeaho, M.-L., Holm, K., and Visakorpi, J. K. (1988). Reticulin antibody, arthritis, and coeliac disease in children. *Lancet*, **i**, 479–480.

[59] Hicklin, J. A., McEwen, L. M., and Morgan, J. E. (1980). The effect of diet on rheumatoid arthritis. *Clin. Allergy*, **10**, 463 (abstract).

[60] Darlington, L. G., Ramsey, N. W., and Mansfield, J. R. (1986). Placebo-controlled, blind study of dietary manipulation therapy in rheumatoid arthritis. *Lancet*, **i**, 236–238.

[61] Stanworth, D. R. (1985). IgA dysfunction in rheumatoid arthritis. *Immunol. Today*, **6**, 43–45.

[62] Green, F. H. Y., and Freed, D. L. J. (1978). Antibody-facilitated digestion and the consequences of its failure. In Hemmings, W. A. (ed.), *Antigen Absorption by the Gut*, MTP Ltd., Lancaster.

[63] Paganelli, R., Atherton, D. J., and Levinsky, R. J. (1983). Differences between normal and milk allergic subjects in their immune responses after milk ingestion. *Arch. Dis. Child.*, **58**, 201–206.

[64] Panush, R. S., Carter, R. L., Katz, P., Kowsari, B., Longley, S., and Finnie, S. (1983). Diet therapy for rheumatoid arthritis. *Arthritis Rheum.*, **26**, 462–471.
Ziff, M. (1983). Diet in the treatment of rheumatoid arthritis. *Arthritis Rheum.*, **26**, 457–461.

[65] Freed, D. L. J. (1985). Lectins. *Br. Med. J.*, **290**, 584–586.

[66] Axford, J. S., Mackenzie, L., Lydyard, P. M., Hay, F. C., Isenberg, D. A., and Roitt, I. M. (1987). Reduced B-cell galactosyltransferase activity in rheumatoid arthritis. *Lancet*, **ii**, 1486–1488.

[67] Concon, J. M., Newberg, D. S., and Eades, S. N. (1983). Lectins in wheat gluten proteins. *J. Agric. Food Chem.*, **31**, 939–941.

[68] Parham, P. (1988). Presentation and processing of antigens in Paris. *Immunol. Today*, **9**, 65–68.

[69] Pujol-Borrell, R., Hanafusa, T., Chiovato, L., and Bottazzo, G. F. (1983). Lectin-induced expression of DR antigen on human cultured follicular thyroid cells. *Nature (London)*, **304**, 71–73.

[70] Winzler, R. J. (1965). Glycoproteins and glycosaminoglycans in plasma and in some other body fluids. In Balazs, E. A., and Jeanloz, R. W. (eds.), *The Amino Sugars*, Vol. IIa, Academic Press, London, pp. 338–352.

[71] Pusztai, A., Clarke, E. M. W., Grant, G., and King, T. P. (1981). The toxicity of *Phaseolus vulgaris* lectins: nitrogen balance and immunochemical studies. *J. Sci. Food Agric.*, **32**, 1037–1046.

[72] Sarkany, I., and Caron, G. A. (1965). Phytohaemagglutinin induced mitotic stimulation of epithelial cells in organ culture of adult human skin. *Br. J. Dermatol.*, **77**, 439–442.

[73] Freed, D. L. J. (1987). Dietary lectins and disease. In Brostoff, J., and Challacombe, S. (eds.), *Food Allergy and Food Intolerance*, Bailliere Tindall, London, pp. 375–400.

[74] Sheldon, P. J., Papamichail, M., and Holborrow, E. J. (1974). Studies on synovial fluid lymphocytes in rheumatoid arthritis. *Ann. Rheum. Dis.*, **33**, 509–514.

[75] Percy, J. S., Davis, P., Russell, A. S., and Brisson, E. (1978). A longitudinal study of *in vitro* tests for lymphocyte function in rheumatoid arthritis. *Ann. Rheum. Dis.*, **37**, 416–420.

[76] Skoldstam, L., Lindstrom, F. D., and Lindblom, B. (1983). Impaired conA suppressor cell activity in patients with rheumatoid arthritis shows normalization during fasting. *Scand. J. Rheumatol.*, **12**, 369–373.

[77] Zuraw, B. L., O'Hair, C. H., Vaughan, J. H., Mathison, D. A., Curd, J. G., and Katz, D. H. (1981). IgE rheumatoid factor in the serum of patients with rheumatoid arthritis, asthma and other diseases. *J. Clin. Invest.*, **68**, 1610–1613.

[78] Sastry-Gollapudi, V. S., and Kind, L. S. (1977). Enhanced reaginic antibody formation to ovalbumin in mice given repeated injections of con A. *Int. Arch. Allergy Appl. Immunol.*, **53**, 569–573.

[79] Astorquiza, M. I., and Sayago, S. (1984). Modulation of IgE response by phytohemagglutinin. *Int. Arch. Allergy Appl. Immunol.*, **73**, 367–369.

[80] Cuong, D. V., Kulcsar, G., Dan, P., Horvath, J., and Nasz, I. (1984). Human adenovirus infection in phytohemagglutinin treated mice. *Acta Microbiol. Hung.*, **31**, 49–53.

[81] Chatterjee, R., Gupta, P., Kashmiri, S. V. S., and Ferrer, J. F. (1985). Phytohemagglutinin activation of the transcription of the bovine leukaemia virus genome requires *de novo* protein synthesis. *J. Virol.*, **54**, 860–863.

[82] Wachter, H., Fuchs, D., Hausen, A., Hengster, P., Reibnegger, G., Reissigl, H., Schoenitzer, D., Schulz, T., Werner, E. R., and Dierich, M. P. (1986). Are conditions linked with T cell stimulation necessary for progressive HTLV-III infection? *Lancet*, **i**, 97.

[83] Carlsson, H. E., Lonngren, J., Goldstein, I. J., Christner, J. E., and Jourdian, G. W. (1976). The interaction of wheat germ agglutinin with keratan from cornea and nasal cartilage. *FEBS Lett.*, **62**, 38–40.

[84] Doi, A., Matsumoto, I., and Seno, N. (1983). Fluorescence studies on the specific interaction between sulfated glycosaminoglycans and potato lectin. *J. Biochem. (Tokyo)*, **93**, 771–775.

[85] Toda, N., Doi, A., Jimbo, A., Matsumoto, I., and Seno, N. (1981). Interaction of sulfated glycosaminoglycans with lectins. *J. Biol. Chem.*, **256**, 5345–5349.

[86] Morris, J. E., and Chan, S. C. (1978). Interactions between chondroitin sulphate and concanavalin A. *Biochim. Biophys. Acta*, **538**, 571–579.

[87] Staprans, I., Felts, J. M., and Butts, R. J. (1983). Quantitative determination of individual glycosaminoglycans in plasma by concanavalin A rocket electrophoresis. *Anal. Biochem.*, **134**, 240–244.

[88] Choi, H. U., Tang, L. H., Johnson, T. L., and Rosenberg, L. (1985). Proteoglycans from bovine nasal and articular cartilages: fractionation of the link proteins by wheat germ agglutinin affinity chromatography. *J. Biol. Chem.*, **260**, 13370–13376.

[89] Baba, T., Takagi, M., and Yagasaki, H. (1985). Ultrastructural cytochemistry of carbohydrates in microfibrils associated with the amorphous elastin in the monkey aorta. *Anat. Rec.*, **213**, 385–391.

[90] Ohno, J., Tajima, Y., and Utsumi, N. (1986). Binding of wheat germ agglutinin in the matrix of rat tracheal cartilage. *Histochem. J.*, **18**, 537–540.

[91] Mallinger, R., Geleff, S., and Bock, P. (1986). Histochemistry of glycosaminoglycans

in cartilage ground substance: Alcian blue staining and lectin-binding affinities in semithin Epon sections. *Histochemistry*, **85**, 121–127.

[92] Wang, T. M., Jee, W. S., Woodbury, L. A., and Matthews, J. L. (1982). Effects of phytohemagglutinin-P (PHA-P) on bone of growing rat. *Metab. Bone Dis. Relat. Res.*, **4**, 193–199.

[93] Popoff, S. N., and Schneider, G. B. (1985). The effects of lectins on the interaction between macrophages and bone *in vitro*. *Cell Tissue Res.*, **241**, 103–109.

[94] Capaldi, M. J., Dunn, M. J., Sewry, C. A., and Dubowitz, V. (1985). Lectin binding in human skeletal muscle: a comparison of 15 different lectins. *Histochem. J.*, **17**, 81–92.

[95] Gaylarde, P. M., and Sarkany, J. (1985). Lectins. *Br. Med. J.*, **290**, 1004.

[96] Farnum, C. E. (1985). Binding of lectin-fluorescein conjugates to intracellular compartments of growth-plate chondrocytes *in situ*. *Am. J. Anat.*, **174**, 419–435.

[97] Itokazu, M., and Tanaka, S. (1985). Localisation of carbohydrate component in human synovial lining cells with fluorescent lectins and enzyme digestion. *Nippon Seikegaka Gakkai Zasshi*, **59**, 1089–1096 (in Japanese; English abstract).

[98] Kelley, R. O., and Lauer, R. B. (1975). On the nature of the external surface of cultured human embryo fibroblasts: an ultrastructural and cytochemical analysis utilising stain and lectin probes. *Differentiation*, **3**, 91–97.

[99] Kouri, T., and Penttinen, R. (1983). Lentil lectin-bound glycoproteins of cultured rheumatoid synovial cells. *Scand. J. Rheumatol.*, **12**, 231–236.

[100] Schumacher, U., and Willershausen, B. (1988). Binding, uptake and effects of lectins on human gingivafibroblasts. In Bøg-Hansen, T. C., and Freed, D. L. J. (eds.), *Lectins, Biology, Biochemistry, Clinical Biochemistry*, Vol. 6, Sigma, St. Louis, pp. 169–176.

[101] Hurum, S., Sodek, J., and Aubin, J. E. (1982). Synthesis of collagen, collagenase and collagenase inhibitors by cloned human gingival fibroblasts and the effect of concanavalin A. *Biochem. Biophys. Res. Commun.*, **107**, 357–366.

[102] Whiteside, T. L., Worrall, J. G., Prince, R. K., Buckingham, R. B., and Rodnan, G. P. (1985). Soluble mediators from mononuclear cells increase the synthesis of glycosaminoglycan by dermal fibroblast cultures derived from normal subjects and progressive systemic sclerosis patients. *Arthritis Rheum.*, **28**, 188–197.

[103] Saklatvala, J., and Sarsfield, S. J. (1982). Lymphocytes induce resorption of cartilage by producing catabolin. *Biochem. J.*, **202**, 275–278.

[104] Wortmann, J., Prinz, R., Ullrich, K., and von Figura, K. (1979). Effect of lectins on the metabolism of sulfated glycosaminoglycans in cultured fibroblasts. *Biochim. Biophys. Acta*, **588**, 26–34.

[105] Rola-Pleszczynski, M., Lieu, H., Hamel, J., and Lemaire, I. (1982). Stimulated human lymphocytes produce a soluble factor which inhibits fibroblast migration. *Cell Immunol.*, **74**, 104–110.

[106] Dayer, J. M. (1982). Aspects of resorption and formation of connective tissue during chronic inflammation in rheumatoid arthritis. *Eur. J. Rheumatol. Inflamm.*, **5**, 457–468.

[107] Anastassiades, T. P., and Wood, A. (1981). Effect of soluble products from lectin-stimulated lymphocytes on the growth, adhesiveness, and glycosaminoglycan synthesis of cultured synovial fibroblastic cells. *J. Clin. Invest.*, **68**, 792–802.

[108] Whiteside, T. L., Buckingham, R. B., Prince, R. K., and Rodnan, G. P. (1984). Products of activated mononuclear cells modulate accumulation of collagen by normal dermal and scleroderma fibroblasts in culture. *J. Lab. Clin. Med.*, **104**, 355–369.

[109] Bräuer, R., Henzgen, S., Thoss, K., and Waldmann, G. (1983). Biphasic changes of the immunological reactivity in the course of experimental lectin-induced arthritis of rabbits. *Exp. Pathol.*, **24**, 117–131.

[110] Prujansky, A., Ravid, A., and Sharon, N. (1978). Cooperativity of lectin binding to lymphocytes and its relevance to mitogenic stimulation. *Biochim. Biophys. Acta*, **508**, 137–146.

[111] Forsdyke, D. R. (1978). Role of complement in the toxicity of dietary legumes. *Med. Hypoth.*, **4**, 97–100.

[112] Ganguly, P., and Fossett, N. G. (1980). Evidence for multiple mechanisms of interaction between wheat germ agglutinin and human platelets. *Biochim. Biophys. Acta*, **627**, 256–261.

[113] Ganguly, P., and Fossett, N. G. (1981). Inhibition of thrombin-induced platelet aggregation by a derivative of wheat germ agglutinin. Evidence for a physiologic

receptor of thrombin in human platelets. *Blood*, **57**, 343–352.

[114] Franz, H. (1988). One hundred years of ricin. In Bøg-Hansen, T. C., and Freed, D. L. J. (eds.), *Lectins: Biology, Biochemistry, Clinical Biochemistry*, Vol. 6, Sigma, St. Louis, MO, pp. 7–13.

[115] Hess, E. V., and Herman, J. H. (1986). Cartilage metabolism and anti-inflammatory drugs in osteoarthritis. *Am. J. Med.*, **81** (Suppl. 5B), 36–64.

[116] Jasin, H. E., and Dingle, J. T. (1981). Human mononuclear cell factors mediate cartilage matrix degradation through chondrocyte activation. *J. Clin. Invest.*, **68**, 571–581.

[117] Hunter, T., Duncan, S., Dew, G., and Reynolds, J. J. (1984). The effect of antirheumatic drugs on the production of collagenase and tissue inhibitor of metalloproteinases (TIMP) by stimulated rabbit articular chondrocytes. *J. Rheumatol.*, **11**, 9–13.

[118] Matsutani, E., and Kuroda, Y. (1982). Effect of lectins on chondrogenesis of cultured quail limb bud cells. *Dev. Biol.*, **89**, 521–526.

[119] Schunke, M., Schumacher, U., and Tillmann, B. (1985). Lectin binding in normal and fibrillated articular cartilage of human patellae. *Virchows Arch. A*, **407**, 221–231.

[120] Bartels, E. M., Danneskiold-Samsøe, B. (1986). Histological abnormalities in muscle from patients with certain types of fibrositis. *Lancet*, **i**, 755–757.

[121] Blau, J. N. (1987). Muscle contraction and tension headache. *Lancet*, **ii**, 222.

[122] Indo, T. (1987). Muscle contraction headache. *Lancet*, **i**, 1370–1371.

[123] Fox, W. W. (1984). *¿La Arthritis—Por que Soportala?*, Plaza y Janes Editores, S.A., Spain.

[124] Rashed, S., Revell, P., Hemingway, A., Low, F., Rainsford, K. and Walker, F. (1989). Effect of non-steroidal anti-inflammatory drugs on the course of osteoarthritis. *Lancet*, Sept 2nd, 519–522.

Index